MW01595887

Instructor's Manual and Testbank to Accompany Essentials of Nursing Research

Methods, Appraisal, and Utilization

Denise F. Polit, PhD

Humanalysis, Inc.
Saratoga Springs, New York
Formerly of the Boston College School of Nursing
Chestnut Hill, Massachusetts

Bernadette P. Hungler, RN, PhD

Boston College School of Nursing
Chestnut Hill, Massachusetts

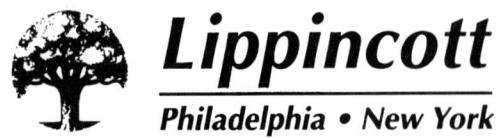

Lippincott

Philadelphia • New York

Fourth Edition

Instructor's Manual and Testbank to Accompany

Essentials of Nursing Research

Methods, Appraisal, and Utilization

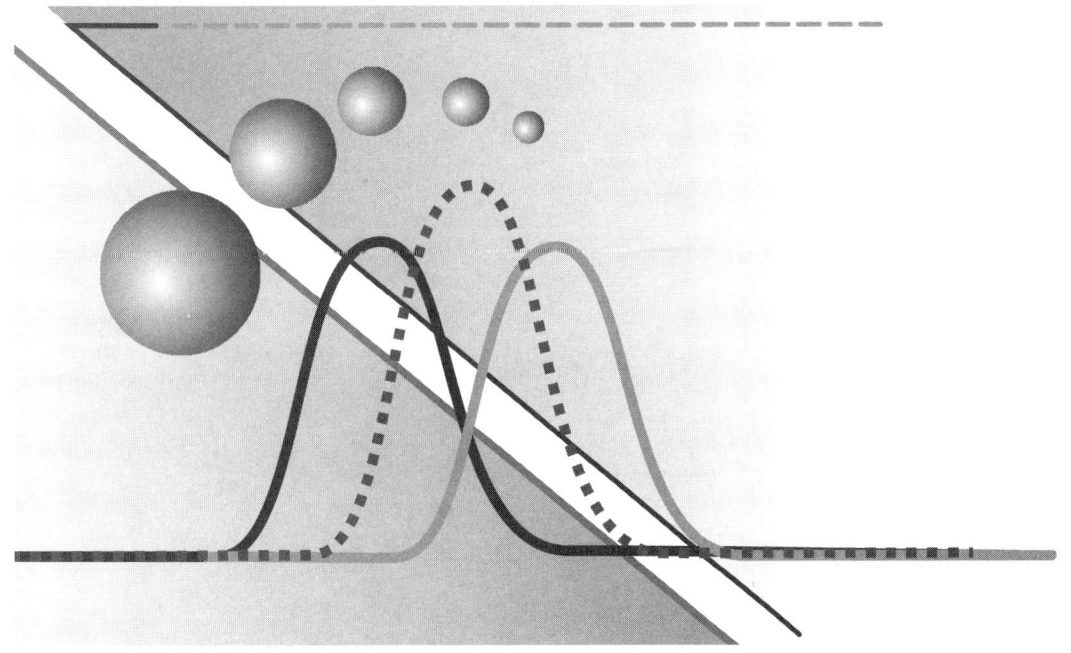

Acquisitions Editor: Margaret Zuccarini
Editorial Assistant: Emily Cotlier
Ancillary Editor: Doris S. Wray
Project Editor: Susan Deitch
Production Manager: Helen Ewan
Production Coordinator: Kathryn Rule
Design Coordinator: Kathy Kelley-Luedtke

Fourth Edition

9 8 7 6 5 4 3 2 1

ISBN: 0-397-55760-4

Care has been taken to confirm the accuracy of the information presented and to describe generally accepted practices. However, the authors, editors, and publisher are not responsible for errors or omissions or for any consequences from application of the information in this book and make no warranty, express or implied, with respect to the contents of the publication.

The authors, editors and publisher have exerted every effort to ensure that drug selection and dosage set forth in this text are in accordance with current recommendations and practice at the time of publication. However, in view of ongoing research, changes in government regulations, and the constant flow of information relating to drug therapy and drug reactions, the reader is urged to check the package insert for each drug for any change in indications and dosage and for added warnings and precautions. This is particularly important when the recommended agent is a new or infrequently employed drug.

Some drugs and medical devices presented in this publication have Food and Drug Administration (FDA) clearance for limited use in restricted research settings. It is the responsibility of the health care provider to ascertain the FDA status of each drug or device planned for use in their clinical practice.

Preface

◩ OVERVIEW

Learning about the techniques of scientific research can be an exceedingly boring and in some cases anxiety-provoking enterprise. There is new jargon to learn, uninteresting details to memorize, intimidating-looking symbols and equations to be confronted, and an impersonal tone and style with which to adapt in reading research reports. In preparing this textbook, we have tried to balance rigorous and factual content with a presentation designed to minimize fears, generate enthusiasm for the research process, and offer concrete support in students' efforts to evaluate and utilize research findings.

We recognize, however, that our role in accomplishing this objective is small relative to your own. We hope that, with the textbook, the Study Guide, and this Instructor's Manual, we are providing you with some basic tools for communicating how research is done, what it can accomplish, and how it can be used. We believe that learning about research methods is analogous to learning how to play a musical instrument: it may be somewhat painful and tedious in the beginning, but it opens up the possibility of a lifetime of growth and rewarding experiences.

The textbook has been written with the needs of the undergraduate student in mind—that is, with the needs of students who are learning how to critically read and appraise the research that others have conducted. It covers the standard content of advanced research methods texts, but in considerably less depth. The length should be manageable in a one-semester course.

Each chapter of the textbook contains explicit guidelines to assist readers in reviewing and critiquing aspects of a research report. Each chapter concludes with a brief description of actual nursing research studies, which students are asked to evaluate. The actual studies that we selected are generally methodologically excellent examples of points that were emphasized in the chapters. In this edition, we have included comments on the actual research examples in this Instructor's Manual.

Our approach to guiding students through important technical features of a study is repeated in the application exercises in the Study Guide. Each of these exercises presents a summary of one or more fictitious studies that illustrates issues discussed in the corresponding chapter. Each example has several limitations (as well as several commendable features) that are incorporated into the example to stimulate discussion of the research methods used. The summary is followed by a series of questions that supplement the textbook's critiquing guidelines, and these questions can be used to provide stucture to classroom discussions. A brief critique of each of these application exercises is included in this Instructor's Manual. The application exercises also contain numerous suggestions of actual research studies amenable to critique by beginning students. In addition, each chapter of this edition of the Study Guide includes fictitious research examples, followed by a critique. The fictitious examples gave us the flexibility to have the "researcher" make noteworthy methodological errors, and to point out those errors in the critique.

Students are told early in the textbook that the design of a research study is a decision-making process—that any research problem can be studied in any number of ways. This theme, repeated throughout the text, is intended to prevent students from believing that because a study is in print, the researchers designed the best possible study. Thus, a major challenge to students is to envision improvements in study design and to recognize the implications of any flaws for interpreting study results. Another equally important challenge is for students to envision using the results of research studies in their own clinical practice—an issue that is discussed at length in the final chapter on research utilization.

◩ SPECIAL COMMENTS ON CHANGES TO THE FOURTH EDITION

This fourth edition represents a fundamental departure from previous editions. In this edition, consistent with trends in nursing research and congruent with the suggestions of several reviewers, qualitative research is given essentially the same degree of coverage in the textbook as quantitative research—and contrasts between the two approaches are repeatedly noted. We believe these revisions represent an important innovation that is unparalleled in research methods textbooks in any discipline.

Like the third edition, this fourth edition reflects our belief that many textbooks fail to sufficiently assist students to learn how to read research reports. We discovered, in preparing the third edition, that many of the terms that are usually considered key terms in research methods textbooks are hardly ever mentioned in research reports—terms such as *dependent* and *independent variable*, for example. We think that intelligent consumers *must* come to understand fundamental research terms, and especially, the concepts they represent. But we also think that beginning students should know what to expect when they turn from a research methods textbook to actual research reports. Throughout this edition, then, we have tried to be especially sensitive in helping students learn how to read research reports and in helping them to make the transition between abstract principles of research methods to concrete studies reported in nursing journals. Thus, a section in each chapter provides tips on "what to expect" in research reports with respect to the topics discussed in that chapter. For example, Chapter 2 explicitly warns students that they may rarely encounter the terms *independent* and *dependent variable* in research reports but that most studies *do* investigate the relationship between independent and dependent variables.

◪ SOME COMMENTS ON THE STUDY GUIDE

We have indicated our purposes in creating an accompanying Study Guide in some detail in the Preface to that book. We have two additional comments to make to instructors using the Study Guide.

First, we do not recommend using the matching exercises and completion exercises as test questions. They were not developed with that purpose in mind. Indeed, many of the items could be challenged as "trick questions" if they were used in a testing situation. We view them as heuristic devices—as an aid to help students review and apply material covered in the textbook. Therefore, we recommend having students perform these exercises in an open-book fashion. We have included answers to these (and some other exercises) in the Instructor's Manual so that instructors can monitor progress, not evaluate performance.

Second, we have filled the Study Guide with hundreds of research possibilities in the hope that they will serve to stimulate the student's imagination. It is our hope that, through the many examples in the textbook and Study Guide, students will appreciate that research ideas do not just "happen," nor are they generated only by scientists working in laboratories. They are created out of curiosity about how the world functions, how human beings behave, and how to improve the kinds of care we give them. Suggestions for research can be developed by anyone, as can ideas about how to incorporate research innovations into the practice of nursing. Skills in research are essential to the conduct of a study, but not to its general conception.

Undergraduate students in particular need to realize that in order to have "facts" and concepts that form the basis of their education, people had to ask questions and seek answers to them. And, people had to evaluate the quality of those answers, which is a skill they should acquire during their course on research methods.

▨ SOME COMMENTS ON THE INSTRUCTOR'S MANUAL

Like the Study Guide, there is a chapter in this manual corresponding to every chapter in the textbook. Each chapter of the manual contains the following:

- *Statement of Intent.* A discussion of the major purposes of the chapter, usually accompanied by our suggestions for what portions merit particular emphasis.
- *Comments on the Actual Research Examples in the Textbook.* High-quality studies invariably were selected as actual research examples in the textbook. Therefore, most of the comments in this Instructor's Manual point out *why,* and in what way, the study is methodologically sound. However, methodologic concerns are also noted.
- *Answers to Selected Study Guide Exercises.* Answers to those questions that have a reasonably objective "right" and "wrong" answer, such as the questions in the matching and completion exercises are presented. (In this edition, these answers also apear in the Appendix to the Study Guide.) Questions that are open-ended and designed to provoke classroom discussion are not dealt with here, except for the critiques of the application exercises.
- *Test Questions and Answers.* A set of multiple choice and true/false questions have been prepared to help you assess students' learning.

We hope that this manual will help you and your students derive a maximally profitable experience from the textbook.

Contents

Instructor's Manual and Testbank to Accompany Essentials of Nursing Research

Methods, Appraisal, and Utilization

Overview of Nursing Research

PART I

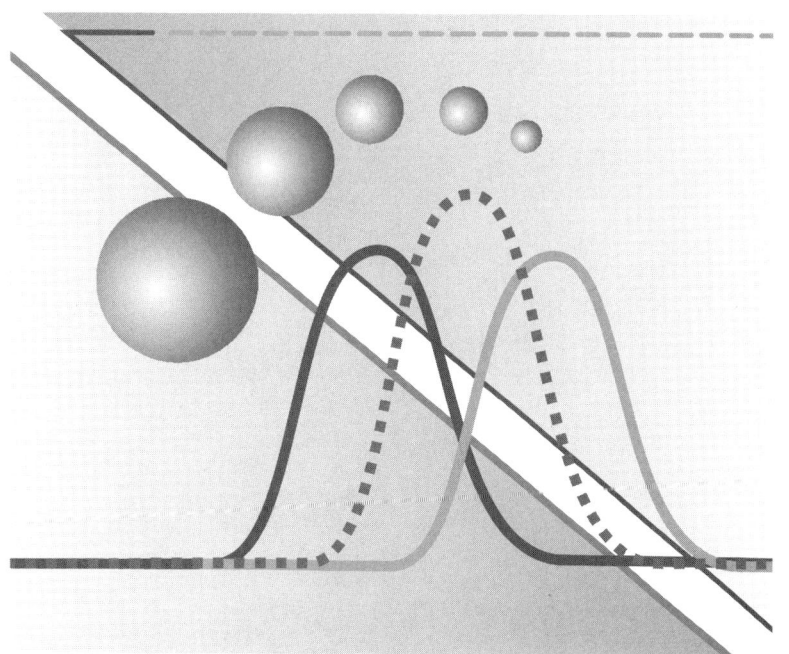

Chapter 1
Introduction to Nursing Research

▧ STATEMENT OF INTENT

A major purpose of this introductory chapter is to establish a foundation for understanding the role of disciplined research in the nursing profession. The chapter provides a brief history of nursing research and discusses the types of problems that nurse researchers have attempted to solve. A fundamental goal of the chapter is to show that research methods have relevance to the practice of nursing. We hope that students will come to appreciate that nursing research is not just for academics; it is for everyone who wants to solve problems or answer questions in a systematic way, and it is also for practicing nurses who must evaluate whether study results should be used as a basis for clinical practice. Chapter 1 discusses the many research-related roles that nurses might adopt along the consumer–producer continuum.

The chapter also presents an overview of the two paradigms (positivist and naturalistic) within which nursing studies are being conducted. It provides a basis for understanding the fundamental philosophical differences between the two paradigms, and links the paradigms to methodologic strategies for acquiring knowledge. Throughout the textbook, distinctions between qualitative and quantitative research are noted, and so it is important for students to grasp the paradigmatic underpinnings of these approaches. The textbook adopts the view that both quantitative and qualitative research have important roles to play in nursing. However, both approaches have limitations, and these should also be understood by students.

▧ COMMENTS ON THE ACTUAL RESEARCH EXAMPLES IN THE TEXTBOOK

Research Example of a Quantitative Study

The study by Okimi and colleagues (1991) is an excellent example of a scientific study undertaken by a team of nurse researchers. Here are a few comments relating to the overall study.

- The study clearly has clinical relevance. As noted by the authors in their discussion section, patient teaching is an inherent, critical part of nursing care, and therefore information about the effects of caffeine for glaucoma patients (or those at risk of glaucoma) is needed.

- The study falls within the positivist paradigm and adheres to a traditional scientific approach. Empirical evidence (*i.e.,* measures of intraocular pressure, or IOP) was collected in a systematic fashion at 1-hour intervals on three consecutive days, using high-quality instrumentation. The researchers controlled for possible biases and contamination by exposing each study participant to all three treatments, in random order. Thus, differences in the IOP of the study participants after treatment could not be the result of random individual differences in IOP, nor of the effects of one treatment in sequence after another. Both individual differences and ordering effects were controlled.

- Appropriately, the study was quantitative. The researchers obtained measures of intraocular pressure (measured as millimeters of mercury [mm Hg]) that were averaged across the three treatments and compared statistically.

- The study has explanation as an implicit goal; that is, the researchers are really interested in answering the question: What causes glaucoma? The more direct purposes of the investigation, however, are prediction and control. The researchers, as a result of their study (especially because the study replicates other research), can tentatively predict that caffeine ingestion will result in increased IOP. Because of this knowledge, the ability to control IOP elevation is enhanced. Full explanation of this phenomenon, however, has not been obtained. The researchers have not ascertained *why* caffeine influences IOP, nor does the study clarify *why* an increase in IOP causes glaucoma.

- Although the study suggests several practical applications (indeed, the authors themselves discuss some of these in their discussion section), the study's aim is more basic than applied.

Research Example of a Qualitative Study

The study by Walcott-McQuigg and co-researchers (1995) is a good example of a culturally sensitive study designed to provide important information on health issues. Here are a few comments relating to the overall study.

- The study is clearly relevant to the practice of nursing. It falls within one of the priority areas established by CORP #1, namely, health promotion. Moreover, it focuses on health issues for a demographic group that has received inadequate research attention in the past.

- The naturalistic paradigm, appropriately, provides the underpinnings for this research. The researchers realized that the dynamic underlying weight control behavior among African American women is complex and poorly understood. To gain insights into the cultural, social, and psychological factors affecting weight in this group, it was essential to talk to some of them directly and to probe deeply into the emotions, values, and beliefs that influence their behavior. It was important for the researcher to understand how these women experienced weight control issues, without imposing any controls or constraints on the research situation.

- The women's emotions and beliefs relating to the cultural and social factors influencing weight control behavior would have been difficult to measure quantitatively. In-depth, qualitative information had the greatest potential to offer insights.
- Like many qualitative studies, this study can be described as exploratory. When a new area is being researched, an exploratory study can provide insights on the full nature and meaning of the phenomenon of interest. An exploratory study can lay the groundwork for more focused research. For example, subsequent studies could examine in a more focused and systematic fashion African American women's cultural values relating to food.
- This study has the potential for applications in the nursing profession, but it did not address or solve an immediate problem. Thus, it lies more on the basic end of the basic–applied continuum.

ANSWERS TO SELECTED STUDY-GUIDE EXERCISES

A.1.

1. a	6. b
2. c	7. c
3. c	8. b
4. c	9. c
5. a	10. d

A.2.

1. a	7. b
2. b	8. d
3. d	9. b
4. a	10. c
5. b	11. a
6. a	12. a

B.

1. Florence Nightingale	9. Scientific
2. Nursing education	10. Empirical
3. 1950s	11. Generalization
4. Clinical practice	12. Reductionist
5. Tradition	13. Field
6. Inductive	14. Quantitative research
7. Determinism	15. Qualitative research
8. Naturalistic	16. Identification

C.7.

a. Basic

b. Applied

c. Applied

d. Basic

e. Basic

f. Applied

g. Basic

h. Applied

D.2. Singleton's study has direct clinical relevance to the practice of nursing. The study is designed to provide information that could be used by other nurses to promote the health and well-being of a vulnerable group, the elderly.

The study adheres to the classical scientific approach, within a positivist tradition. Singleton was attempting to gain systematic knowledge about the effect of alternative techniques of persuasion on the behavior of elderly citizens through direct empirical observation. She controlled the situation by sending half the members of the senior citizens center a positively worded message (*i.e.*, stressing the health benefits of a flu shot) and the other half a negatively worded message (*i.e.*, stressing the health risks of failure to get a flu shot). The behavior of interest, whether the person comes forward for a flu shot, will be directly observable by the researcher. Because the alternative letters were mailed to the elderly impartially (*i.e.*, an elderly person was equally likely to be sent a negatively worded as a positively worded letter) and because the letters were similar in other respects (*e.g.*, both groups were advised of the free transportation and immunizations), we can conclude that the research was characterized by a fairly high degree of control. Although Singleton was observing the behavioral responses of 500 specific elderly citizens, she is presumably interested in generalizing the results more broadly so that others could adopt the most effective strategy for encouraging preventive health practices among the elderly.

As described here, Singleton's study appears not to have an explanatory purpose. At the end of the research, she may learn that one type of communication approach is better than the other, but she will not know *why*. This study appears to have primarily a predictive and control intent (*e.g.*, health care workers could, in the future, predict that a certain approach is more likely to yield high rates of compliance and might want to control subsequent campaigns accordingly).

Singleton's research is applied in nature. She presumably wanted information that would be helpful in developing communication strategies or health care policies for the elderly. This is essentially a utilitarian function.

The basic research question concerns *how many* of the elderly in the two groups came forward to receive a flu shot, and therefore quantitative information was needed. The difference in rates of coming forward would be analyzed using quantitative (statistical) procedures. It is important to note, however, that the study might well be enhanced through the collection of some qualitative information as well. For example, the researcher could contact noncompliers from both groups to ask them if they understood the content of the letter and to seek their general reaction to the message. These people could also be asked why they did not come to the clinic for a flu shot. Thus, even studies that have a positivist framework can sometimes be enhanced by questions that are associated with a naturalistic perspective.

D.3. Rimmer's study delved into an intensely personal and complex area of human experience, and an area that has not yet been carefully researched. Individuals who have lost a parent to a genetically linked disease must develop effective strategies for assessing and managing risk. Health care professionals can perhaps facilitate risk management if they better understand the risk experience from the perspective of those who are experiencing it. Thus, Rimmer's study has the potential to be clinically significant.

The nature of the research problem is well suited to an in-depth examination of the risk experience *as it is lived*—not as it is perceived or appraised by others. What the researcher wanted to study was the people's own interpretations of their experiences, and the researcher sought to obtain this knowledge by letting the individuals speak at length in their own words. By taping the interviews, the researcher was able to capture those words without having to take detailed notes, which can slow down and constrain the interview flow. Given the probing nature of the inquiry, the collection of narrative, subjective information was appropriate.

As suggested by the summary of the study, the researcher's purpose was both descriptive (what are the dimensions of the risk experience?) and exploratory (what is the full nature of the risk experience?). The study appears to be seeking knowledge primarily for knowledge's own sake (*i.e.,* has a basic orientation), but it is not difficult to envision the uses to which that knowledge could be placed.

▨ TEST QUESTIONS AND ANSWERS

Multiple Choice

1. Which of the following groups would be *best* served by the development of a scientific base for nursing practice?
    - a. Nursing administrators
    - b. Nursing educators
    - c. Nursing practitioners
    - *d. Nursing's clientele

2. An especially important goal for the nursing profession is to:
    - a. Conduct research to better understand supply and demand for nurses
    - *b. Establish a scientific base of knowledge for the improvement of practice
    - c. Document the role nursing serves in society
    - d. Establish research priorities

3. Which of the following is *not* a current priority for clinical nursing research?
    - a. Cost-effective health care delivery systems
    - b. Health promotion
    - *c. Nurses' personalities
    - d. Assessment of interventions for people with chronic illness

4. Most nursing studies at mid-century focused on:

    a. Consumer satisfaction

    b. Clinical problems

    c. Health promotion

    *d. Nursing education

5. Which of the following topics most closely conforms to the priorities that have been suggested for future nursing research?

    a. Attitudes of nursing students toward smoking

    *b. Factors associated with patient compliance with treatment

    c. Nursing staff morale and turnover

    d. Number of doctorally prepared nurses in various clinical specialties

6. Deductive reasoning is the process of:

    a. Verifying assumptions

    *b. Developing specific predictions from general principles

    c. Empirically testing observations

    d. Forming generalizations from specific observations

7. To those espousing a naturalistic paradigm, the ontological assumption is that:

    a. A fixed reality exists in nature for humans to understand

    b. The nature of reality has changed over time

    *c. Reality is multiply constructed and multiply interpreted by humans

    d. Reality cannot be studied empirically

8. To those espousing a positivist paradigm, the epistemological assumption is that:

    *a. The researcher is objective and independent of those being studied

    b. The researcher cannot interact with those being studied.

    c. The researcher instructs those being studied to be objective in providing information

    d. The distance between the researcher and those being researched is minimized to enhance the interactive process

9. The traditional scientific approach is *not* characterized by which of the following attributes?

    a. Control over external factors

    b. Systematic measurement and observation of natural phenomena

    c. Logical reasoning

    *d. Emphasis on a holistic view of a phenomenon, studied in a rich context

10. Empiricism refers to:

    a. Making generalizations from specific observations

    b. Deducing specific predictions from generalizations

    *c. Gathering evidence rooted in objective reality

    d. Verifying the assumptions on which the study was based

11. A hallmark of the scientific approach is that it is:
  a. Infallible
  b. Holistic
  *c. Systematic
  d. Flexible

12. Which of the following limits the power of the scientific approach to answer questions about human life?
  a. The necessity of departing from traditional beliefs
  *b. The difficulty of measuring psychosocial characteristics of humans
  c. The inability to control potential biases
  d. The shortage of theories about human behavior

13. The scientific approach has its intellectual roots in:
  *a. Logical positivism
  b. Determinism
  c. Phenomenology
  d. Inductive reasoning

14. One of the criticisms of the scientific approach is that it is overly:
  a. Logical
  b. Deterministic
  c. Empirical
  *d. Reductionist

15. Naturalistic qualitative research typically:
  a. Involves deductive processes
  b. Attempts to control the research context to better understand the nature of the phenomenon being studied
  *c. Takes place in the field
  d. Focuses on the idiosyncrasies of those being studied

16. Quantitative and qualitative research do *not* share which of the following features?
  a. A desire to gain an understanding of the true state of human affairs
  *b. Roots in 19th century phenomenological thought
  c. Reliance on external evidence collected through the senses
  d. Utility to the nursing profession

17. A descriptive question that a qualitative researcher might ask is:
  *a. What are the dimensions of this phenomenon?
  b. How frequently does this phenomenon occur?
  c. What is the average duration of this phenomenon?
  d. How prevalent is this phenomenon?

18. A researcher wants to investigate the effect of patients' body position on blood pressure. The study would most likely be:
  a. Qualitative
  *b. Quantitative
  c. Inductive
  d. Insufficient information to determine

19. A researcher wants to study the process by which people make decisions about seeking treatment for infertility. The researcher's paradigmatic orientation most likely is:
    a. Positivism   c. Empiricism
    b. Determinism   *d. Naturalism

20. A researcher is studying the effect of massage on the alleviation of pain in cancer patients. The study would be described as:
    a. Descriptive   *c. Applied
    b. Exploratory   d. Basic

True/False

(F)   1. Throughout the history of nursing research, most studies have focused on clinical problems.

(F)   2. The journal *Nursing Research* began publication during the early 1900s.

(T)   3. Most people would agree that nursing research began with Florence Nightingale.

(F)   4. Nursing practice currently has a strong scientific base.

(F)   5. The current trend in nursing research is a focus on nursing administration.

(F)   6. The journal *Nursing Research* is currently the only major journal for communicating the results of nursing research studies.

(T)   7. Journal clubs for practicing nurses involve meetings to discuss and critically evaluate research studies.

(F)   8. All producers of nursing research work in universities and schools of nursing.

(F)   9. Deductive reasoning is the process of developing generalizations from specific observations.

(T)   10. A paradigm is a general perspective on the nature of the real world.

(T)   11. According to the positivist paradigm, there is an objective reality that can be understood by researchers.

(F)   12. The naturalistic paradigm is associated with structured, quantitative research.

(T)   13. A naturalistic researcher attempts to understand rather than control the context of those being studied.

(F)   14. Nursing leaders currently are suggesting that in-depth, process-oriented studies are more important than controlled quantitative studies for nursing practice.

(F)   15. Empirical evidence is information derived from introspective analysis of real-world phenomena.

(T)   16. The scientific approach assumes that all phenomena have antecedent causes.

(T)   17. Quantitative researchers are more likely than qualitative researchers to pursue research with prediction and control as a purpose.

(F)   18. Quantitative researchers tend to emphasize the dynamic and holistic aspects of human experience.

(T)   19. Applied research is designed to solve immediate problems.

(F)   20. Research questions that focus on identification (*e.g.*, What is this phenomenon?) are most likely to be applied in nature.

Chapter 2
Overview of the Research Process

◼ STATEMENT OF INTENT

The purpose of Chapter 2 is to provide students with some basic groundwork for dealing with the remainder of the text. There are three main parts to this chapter. The first part introduces research terminology that recurs throughout the text. The students' firm grounding in basic research terms should facilitate their ability to grasp more complex methodologic concepts later in the book and to begin to read research reports. This edition also distinguishes the basic terminology used by qualitative and quantitative researchers—for example, *subject* versus *informant.* A chart summarizing differences in terminology has been included.

The second part of the chapter provides an overview of the steps that a researcher undertakes in conducting a research study. Separate sections are devoted to describing the general progression of activities in qualitative and quantitative studies.

The final section offers some practical assistance in reading research reports. Because the research literature (especially for quantitative studies) is sometimes anxiety provoking to students because of its jargon, its dense and impersonal language, and its presentation of statistical information, they may need assistance in overcoming their aversion to reading research reports. It is probably best to encourage students to read research reports somewhat superficially at first to get the gist of the report—that is, to understand what the basic story is—without worrying about technical details. A class "translation" of a research report might be a useful exercise.

COMMENTS ON THE ACTUAL RESEARCH EXAMPLES IN THE TEXTBOOK

Research Example of a Quantitative Study

The textbook provided a brief abstract of some aspects of a study by Tuten and Gueldner (1991). The study compared the effectiveness of using a sodium chloride versus a dilute heparin solution for maintaining peripheral intermittent intravenous devices (PIIDs). Here are a few comments about that study, with specific reference to the concepts discussed in Chapter 2.

- Given the nature of the research question, a quantitative approach was appropriate. Incidence of device complications, the dependent variable, is easily measured and quantified.
- This was an unusual research report in that it explicitly labeled the independent variables and dependent variables. The study was about the *relationship* between type of solution for PIID maintenance (the independent variable) and patency and complications (the dependent variables). Note that, like many studies, this one had multiple dependent variables.
- Type of solution was a created (not an attribute) variable. The researchers actively intervened to maintain some subjects' PIIDs with one type of solution and other subjects' PIIDs with the other. Type of solution is a categorical variable.
- Operational definitions of the dependent variables were not fully elaborated in the report, although it does appear that a complete specification was provided to those who collected the data on the PIID Complication Assessment Form. The absence of the full operational definitions in the report could simply reflect space constraints in the journal. (Note that the data were collected by staff nurses, not by researchers.)
- The study purpose mentions a dependent variable (patency) that was not specified by the researchers in their statement of what the dependent variables were.
- The report conformed fairly closely to a standard structure for a journal research report.

Research Example of a Qualitative Study

A brief overview of an interesting study by Langner (1993) was included in the textbook. A few comments on aspects of this study discussed in Chapter 2 follow:

- The phenomenon under study was a complex, dynamic process—the process of managing the caregiving of an elderly relative. Although there has been considerable research on caregivers in recent years, relatively little has focused on day-to-day experiences and processes over time.

- Because so little prior work had focused on the day-to-day experiences of caregivers, a qualitative study was appropriate. Langner did not know in advance what the caregiving process would be like—nor how many concepts would evolve. She allowed the key concepts to emerge during the course of the interviews. Only after analyzing her data did Langner discovery that three central strategies were adopted to manage the caregiving process.
- There were no concepts in this study that could be described as "independent" or "dependent" variables. Nor, as is appropriate for qualitative studies, were there operational definitions of any variables.
- Given Langner's interest in describing a *process*, it was appropriate to collect data from her study participants on several occasions over an extended period. This allowed changes in adaptation to caregiving to unfold.
- In describing the three central processes in her report, Langner included examples of *raw data*—that is, excerpts from interviews that exemplified the themes that emerged.
- Although the excerpt in the textbook does not present this information, students who have read the entire research report may have noted that the researcher did examine patterns of association with regard to the nature of the kinship relationship (*e.g.,* spouse, sibling, parent–child, etc.). The author noted that the kinship role was not associated with differences in the caregiving process: "Whereas the respondents in the present study represented a variety of kinship relationships and often had competing familial, social, or professional responsibilities, there was no evidence to support a qualitative difference among the respondents' perceptions of their duties and responsibilities or of the strategies they used to meet the challenges of caregiving" (p. 591).
- The organization of the report followed fairly closely a traditional format, except that the introduction was divided into distinct subsections, which is not always the case.

▨ ANSWERS TO SELECTED STUDY-GUIDE EXERCISES

A.1.
1. a	5. b
2. c	6. a
3. b	7. c
4. a	8. c

A.2.
1. a	3. c
2. b	4. b

5. a   9. a
6. a   10. b
7. b   11. a
8. c   12. b

A.3.

1. b   5. b
2. c   6. c
3. b   7. c
4. a   8. c

B.

1. Principal investigator,   15. Qualitative, quantitative
   project director   16. Quantitative
2. Subjects, study participants   17. Research design
3. Concepts   18. Sample
4. Variable   19. Empirical (data collection)
5. Categorical   20. Data analysis
6. Independent   21. Pilot study
7. Dependent   22. Research report, journal
8. Independent   articles
9. Data   23. Dissemination
10. Operational definitions   24. Gaining entrée
11. Qualitative   25. Saturation
12. Patterns of association   26. Abstract, introduction, method,
13. Causal (cause and effect)   results, discussion, references
14. Functional

C. 3 and C.4.*

Independent   ### *Dependent*

a. Participation/nonparticipation in   Nursing effectiveness (continu-
   assertiveness training (categori-   ous)
   cal)

b. Patients' postural positioning (cat- Respiratory function (continuous)
   egorical)

c. Amount of touch by nursing staff   Patients' psychological well-being
   (continuous)   (continuous)

---

*For some of these variables, there is no absolutely correct answer with regard to whether the variable is categorical or continuous because it would depend on the operational definition established by the researcher. For example, in Question C.3(n), the educational backgrounds of women could be measured as a continuous variable (number of years of schooling completed), or as a categorical variable (did not complete high school versus completed high school). Because researchers can always collapse continuous variables into categorical variables, we have indicated those variables that *could* be continuous as continuous variables.

d. Frequency of turning patients (continuous)

Incidence of decubitus (continuous)

e. Educational preparation of nurses (categorical)

Turnover rate (continuous)

f. Patients' age (continuous) and gender (categorical)

Tolerance for pain (continuous)

g. Number of prenatal visits (continuous)

Labor and delivery outcomes (continuous—*e.g.,* length of time in labor; or categorical—*e.g.,* vaginal versus cesarean delivery)

h. Pediatric versus adult intensive care unit (ICU) assignment (categorical)

Nurses' stress levels (continuous)

i. Student nurses' clinical grades (continuous)

On-the-job performance (continuous)

j. Method of preoperative teaching (categorical)

Anxiety levels of patients (continuous)

k. Level of participation in continuing education activities (continuous)

Nurses' promotions (categorical)

l. Time of day (continuous)

Hearing acuity among the elderly (continuous)

m. Congruity of nurses' and patients' cultural backgrounds (categorical)

Patient satisfaction with nursing care (continuous)

n. Women's educational backgrounds (continuous)

Breast self-examination practices (categorical)

o. Setting of childbirth: home versus hospital (categorical)

Parents' satisfaction with childbirth experience (continuous)

D.2. In Hebert's fictitious study, the nature of the patient's home environment was the independent variable, and reaction to hospital noise was the dependent variable. As defined, type of home environment was a continuous variable because number of household members can range on a continuum from 1 to some very large number. The dependent variable was categorical: a patient either was or was not dissatisfied with hospital noise levels.

Hebert's operational definitions could be improved. For the home environment variable, it would be possible for anyone to replicate the measurements according to the definition given. However, for the dependent variable (reaction to hospital noise), further specification is needed: we do not know what the five questions were and how they were scored; we also do not know the basis for dividing subjects into satisfied or dissatisfied groups.

More important, Hebert's definitions were probably not as well conceptualized as possible. For example, for the independent variable, it seems advisable to add dimensions other than quantity of household members as measures of the home environment. Examples include the presence versus absence of children younger than age 10, the proportion of minors to adults in the household, the crowdedness of the household (*e.g.,* number of people divided by the number of rooms), and the number of televisions and radios in the household.

The dependent variable, too, could probably have been defined better or defined in alternative ways. One of the problems with the current definition is that it depends on subjects' recall at discharge rather than on patients' immediate reactions to noises. In addition to obtaining self-reports during hospitalization, Hebert could have had nurses record the number of patient complaints about noise levels.

One can imagine a causal *pathway* between the two variables: number of household members might affect people's tolerance for different noise levels, and hence their satisfaction with hospital noises. However, it cannot really be said that number of household members *causes* dissatisfaction with noise levels. In fact, it cannot even be assumed that number of household members *influences* the patient's reaction to noise. It might be that people who are generally more comfortable in an environment with a lot of activity and noise seek to establish larger households (*e.g.,* they might have more children). In other words, there are a number of possible explanations for a relationship between household size and noise tolerance. The relationship would best be characterized as functional.

Aspects with the home environment and people's reactions to noise can be quantified, and hence a quantitative study is not inappropriate. However, we can also envision that an in-depth, qualitative look at the home environments of patients with different hospital experiences could also be profitable—and might suggest to a quantitative researcher the aspects of the home environment that are especially likely to be related to tolerance for hospital noise.

D.4. The general phenomenon that Weiser focused on was patients' views about the meaning of noncompliance with a therapeutic regimen. There are no "independent" and "dependent" variables in this investigation. Weiser was not interested in what caused or influenced the patients' viewpoints, nor on what the consequences of those viewpoints were. Rather, the researcher wanted to obtain personalized, subjective accounts of what noncompliance meant in the lives of chronically ill people. Such a focus is appropriate for a qualitative researcher.

The brief summary presented in the Study Guide does not discuss whether the researcher examined patterns of association. Weiser would not have known in advance (nor do we know from the description) whether interesting patterns might emerge—indeed, the point of an exploratory qualitative study is to let the data speak for themselves. However, it is very well possible that interesting patterns would have been detected and explored by the researcher. For example, one can imagine that men and women might have different viewpoints about compliance; the *nature* of the chronic illness might also play a role in the meaning of noncompliance.

Given that the study focused on a rural population, Weiser's decision to recruit study participants through a health clinic was probably a reasonable one.

However, it might have been advisable to conduct the in-depth interviews in the settings in which noncompliance typically occurs—in the homes of the participants, rather than in the clinic itself.

▨ TEST QUESTIONS AND ANSWERS

Multiple Choice

1. Which of the following terms is *not* typically used by quantitative researchers to refer to people who participate in a study?
   - *a. Informant
   - b. Respondent
   - c. Study participant
   - d. Subject

2. Which of the following terms is used by both qualitative and quantitative researchers to refer to an abstraction under study?
   - *a. Concept
   - b. Construct
   - c. Phenomenon
   - d. Variable

3. "Male" is:
   - *a. Not a variable
   - b. A categorical variable
   - c. An active variable
   - d. A continuous variable

4. Of the following, the most appropriate example of an attribute variable is:
   - a. Shift assignment
   - b. Method of teaching
   - c. Nurse–client teaching
   - *d. Blood type

5. "Pulse rate" is:
   - a. Not a variable
   - b. A categorical variable
   - c. Inherently an independent variable
   - *d. None of the above

6. "Nursing effectiveness" is:
   - a. A concept
   - b. A construct
   - c. A variable
   - *d. All of the above

7. The dependent variable(s) in the research question, "Is the job performance of nurses affected by salary or perceived job autonomy?" is (are):
   - *a. Job performance
   - b. Salary
   - c. Perceived job autonomy
   - d. Both salary and perceived job autonomy

8. The independent variable in the research question, "What is the effect of noise levels on postoperative pain or blood pressure fluctuations in ICU patients?" is:
   - a. Blood pressure
   - b. ICU patients
   - *c. Noise levels
   - d. Postoperative pain

9. The independent variable in the hypothesis, "Baccalaureate degree–prepared nurses will practice more rehabilitative nursing measures on a client in an ICU than will associate degree–prepared nurses" is:

    a. Associate degree–prepared nurses

    b. Baccalaureate degree–prepared nurses

    c. Rehabilitative nursing measures

    *d. Type of educational background of nurse

10. The purpose of an operational definition in a quantitative study is to:

    a. Assign numeric values to variables

    *b. Specify how a variable will be defined and measured

    c. State the expected relationship between the variables under investigation

    d. Designate the overall plan by which the data will be collected

11. Which of the following is a datum from a quantitative research study on the labor and delivery experiences of women older than age 40?

    a. Length of time in labor

    *b. 107 oz

    c. Infant's Apgar score

    d. Vaginal versus cesarean delivery

12. Which of the following is a datum from a qualitative research study on the labor and delivery experiences of women older than age 40?

    a. 14.6 hours in labor

    b. 60-minute interviews one day after delivery

    *c. "It was a lot more painful than I ever imagined."

    d. 15 primiparous women with a vaginal delivery

13. For which of the following pairs of variables is there most likely to be a relationship that could be described as causal?

    *a. Degree of physical activity–heart rate

    b. Stress–coping style

    c. Age–health beliefs

    d. Parity—postpartum depression

14. A researcher's expectations about the outcomes of a quantitative study are generally expressed in the form of a:

    *a. Hypothesis

    b. Theory

    c. Criterion variable

    d. Research problem

15. The overall plan developed by the researcher to obtain answers to the questions being studied is called the:

    a. Coding plan

    b. Proposal

    c. Problem statement

    *d. Research design

16. The individuals who provide data in a research investigation are collectively referred to as the:

    a. Research producers

    b. Population

    *c. Sample

    d. Assistants

17. A qualitative researcher typically makes a lot of decisions about data collection and the research sample:

    a. While reviewing the literature
    b. During the development of a research proposal
    *c. While the study is in progress in the field
    d. After a pilot study has been conducted

18. Nurses are most likely to find research results in:

    a. Poster sessions
    *b. Journal articles
    c. Books
    d. Dissertations

19. In a research report, a review of prior research on the problem under study is most likely to be found in the

    *a. Introduction
    b. Methods section
    c. Results section
    d. Discussion section

20. In which section of a research report would the following sentence most likely be found: "The data showed a four-phase process of parental adaptation to the death of a child."

    a. Introduction
    b. Methods
    *c. Results
    d. Discussion

True/False

(T)   1. The term *subject* is used primarily in quantitative research.

(F)   2. Quantitative researchers focus on concrete concepts, whereas qualitative researchers study abstract constructs.

(F)   3. Body temperature is an example of a constant.

(T)   4. Body weight is more heterogeneous among all adults in Boston than it is among Bostonians who belong to a weight-loss program.

(F)   5. An attribute variable is one that the researcher creates for research purposes.

(T)   6. Blood pressure is an example of a continuous variable.

(F)   7. The independent variable is the one that the researcher is interested in explaining.

(F)   8. Variables are inherently either dependent or independent.

(F)   9. In a study of the health care needs of African Americans in urban versus rural areas, race would be the independent variable.

(T) 10. An operational definition specifies the procedures and tools required for measurement of a concept.

(F) 11. In a study of the effectiveness of massage in reducing the pain of oncology patients, the researcher is investigating a functional relationship.

(T) 12. The relationship between infants' length and weight at birth is an example of a functional relationship.

(T) 13. Quantitative research typically involves a fairly linear progression of tasks.

(F) 14. The plan for converting verbal information into numeric form is known as the research design.

(T) 15. If the population of interest were all RNs in the United States, a sample of nurses consisting entirely of women would not be representative.

(F) 16. The final phase in a research project is the analytic phase.

(F) 17. Raw data are rarely presented in qualitative research reports.

(F) 18. Qualitative and quantitative researchers always perform a literature review before collecting their data to learn what the state-of-the-art is.

(F) 19. In a qualitative study, sample size decisions are usually determined on the basis of the number of informants available in the setting.

(T) 20. Peer reviewers of a nursing research report are usually nurse researchers.

(T) 21. An abstract of a journal article appears at the beginning of the report.

(T) 22. The research design for a study is usually described in the Methods section of a research report.

(F) 23. A statistical test is used in quantitative studies to prove that the study was significant.

(T) 24. The discussion section of a research report usually includes an interpretation of the results and comments on their implications.

(F) 25. Novice research consumers have difficulty reading research reports primarily because they have an insufficient knowledge base on the topic under investigation.

Preliminary Steps in the Research Process

PART II

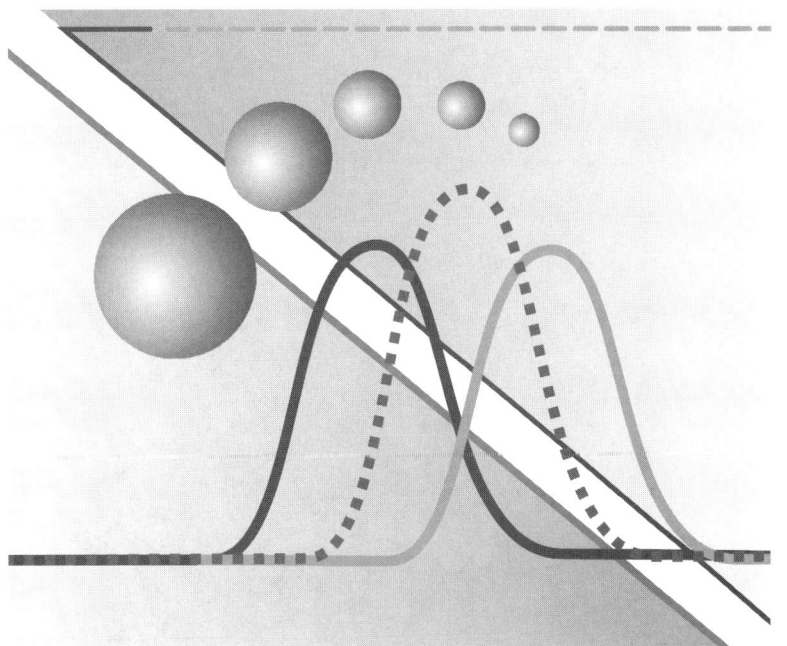

Chapter 3
Research Problems, Research Questions, and Hypotheses

◪ STATEMENT OF INTENT

Chapter 3 discusses methods of articulating and communicating information about the research problem through statements of purpose, research questions, and research hypotheses. There is some inconsistency in research textbooks concerning the aims, goals, purposes, and objectives of research, and the first section of the chapter explains how these and other related terms are used in this textbook. A graphic example presented in Table 3-1 should help to clarify how the terms are defined.

The chapter then describes some of the origins of research ideas and examines the process of narrowing a specific problem from a general topic of interest. The issue of problem development within the two major paradigms is described. Alternative ways of wording the problem statement are also described, and differences between research questions and statements of purpose are discussed. This chapter also provides guidance to beginning research consumers on how to *find* a problem statement in a research report and on how to evaluate it (substantively and methodologically) once it is located.

The next part of the chapter focuses on hypotheses. The chapter explains the role that hypotheses play in giving direction to a quantitative study and in explicitly communicating that direction. It argues that quantitative studies, except for ones that are purely descriptive, generally profit from the development of hypotheses before data collection. The chapter also describes the characteristics of workable hypotheses and provides guidance for a critical evaluation of hypotheses appearing in research reports. Because the wording of hypotheses is often problematic to students, considerable attention is paid to the issue of alternative wordings. The important point is that hypotheses must make predictions about the *relationship* between two (or more) variables.

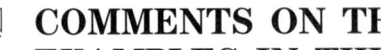 COMMENTS ON THE ACTUAL RESEARCH EXAMPLES IN THE TEXTBOOK

Research Example from a Quantitative Study

Matthews's (1991) presentation of her research problem had a number of positive features as well as a few limitations. Here are some comments relating to the researcher's description of her purpose, research questions, and hypothesis.

- Although Matthews's problem statement was not placed early in the report, a separate, easily located section was devoted to it. This section included the statement of purpose and, under separate subsections, the hypotheses and research questions. The section was logically placed after the author's review of the literature, in which a need for the research was documented. (The literature review section concluded as follows: "Few studies, however, have addressed the effects of neonates' feeding behavior difficulties on the mother and her motivation to continue breastfeeding.")
- The statement of purpose clearly indicated the research variables and the population of interest. The statement of purpose suggested, through the use of the verb "to determine," a well-focused study that would use quantitative methods of data collection. This is consistent with the actual conduct of the study.
- The hypothesis was well worded: it stated an expected relationship between the independent (neonates' feeding behaviors) and dependent (mothers' satisfaction) variables; it indicated the population of interest (mothers with neonates); and it even indicated how the independent variable would be operationalized (scores on the Infant Breastfeeding Assessment Tool), although it did not provide comparable information for the dependent variable.
- The hypothesis flowed directly from the statement of purpose and appears to be consistent with existing theory and research on this topic.
- The four research questions are all related to the theme of maternal breastfeeding satisfaction, but they are not all linked directly to the statement of purpose. The first question is a purely descriptive one; it asks about the incidence of maternal satisfaction and dissatisfaction with breastfeeding. The second question is essentially a rewording of the statement of purpose in the interrogative form and therefore seems redundant and unnecessary, especially in light of the fact that a formal hypothesis has also been stated. The third research question has the potential of being a good subproblem; it asks if there are factors that distinguish between different groups of mothers. However, this research question as stated is somewhat ambiguous, at two levels. First, it does not make clear whether the author was interested in differences in mothers with different levels of satisfaction or in differences in mothers whose neonates have different breastfeeding competence (we later learn that Matthews's interest was in differences in ma-

ternal satisfaction). Second, it does not make explicit the factors that will be explored to differentiate the mothers. In the Results section, we learn that Matthews examined such factors as parity and use of medication during labor. The fourth question is similarly ambiguous; Matthews gives us no clue in the question itself regarding what types of "other effects" on the mothers she might be interested in examining. A subsequent section indicates that the author was primarily interested in exploring in a qualitative way such effects as maternal frustration and anxiety. Thus, some of the research questions could have been more clearly stated. Additionally, the statement of purpose could be modified slightly to be more inclusive of the full range of the researcher's interest. One possibility might be the following: The purpose of this study was to explore maternal satisfaction with breastfeeding and to determine whether satisfaction was affected by neonate breastfeeding competence and by other factors such as parity and use of medication during labor.

Research Example from a Qualitative Study

Artinian (1995) conducted a study on "special relationships" between nurses and cancer patients. Here are a few comments regarding Artinian's description of her study purpose:

- Artinian focused on a topic that is central to the practice of nursing, namely, the helping relationship. She narrowed this general problem area to a focus on relationships in which intense involvement developed. Thus, the scope was appropriately delimited.
- The problem was well suited to an intensive, in-depth approach that is characteristic of qualitative studies. The approach had special potential to be productive because, as the researcher noted, existing research had never systematically examined the *process* by which nurse/patient pairs develop special relationships.
- Artinian communicated both a general statement of purpose, as well as more specific research questions. Both the statement of purpose and research questions were clearly worded—although the research questions could have benefited from a reference to the type of patients (cancer patients) under study, and the nature of the setting for the investigation (cancer units). The information was communicated early in the report to assist readers in understanding immediately what the study was about.
- Consistent with the fact that this was a qualitative investigation that aimed primarily to *describe* and *explore* special relationships between nurses and patients, there were no research hypotheses being tested. However, it should be noted that another researcher might well develop hypotheses about special relationships based on Artinian's findings and test those hypotheses in a new study.

ANSWERS TO SELECTED STUDY-GUIDE QUESTIONS

A.1.

1. b
2. c
3. a
4. b
5. a
6. c
7. b
8. a

A.2.

1. a
2. c
3. d
4. a
5. b
6. d
7. a
8. c
9. b
10. d
11. b
12. c
13. b
14. a
15. c

B.

1. Research problem
2. Research question
3. Research aims, objectives
4. Experience, literature, social issues, theory, external sources
5. Qualitative
6. Unfeasible
7. Unresearchable
8. Introduction
9. Relationship
10. Two
11. Multivariate (complex)
12. Null (statistical)

C.6

	Independent	***Dependent***
4a.	Clinical specialty area	Attitudes toward mental retardation
4b.	Nurses versus patients	Perceived importance of attending to physical versus emotional needs
4c.	Type of Nursing Care (primary versus team nursing)	Patient satisfaction with nursing care
4d.	Frequency of turning	Incidence of decubitus ulcers
4e.	Type of nursing preparation (baccalaureate versus associate program)	Use of therapeutic touch
5a.	Number of prior blood donations	Stress
5b.	Nurses' frequency of initiating conversation	Patients' ratings of nursing effectiveness

5c. Patients' ratings of nurses' informativeness	Degree of preoperative stress
5d. Draining versus no draining of peritoneum	Incidence of infection
5e. Method of delivery (cesarean versus vaginal)	Incidence of postpartum depression

D.2. Clain's hypotheses are fairly clearly stated and are logically derived from the problem statement initially posed by the researcher. There is, nevertheless, some room for improvement. The first hypothesis is the most problematic. As stated, it is not directly testable by scientific methods because there is no relationship to test. There is only one variable, the frequency of referring to nursing notes on patients' charts. What criteria will Clain use to determine what is infrequent? It would have been more appropriate to drop the first hypothesis and to state that, in addition to testing the other hypotheses, one of the purposes of the study was to *describe* the frequency with which nursing notes are reviewed by hospital personnel. Alternatively, the first hypothesis could have been modified to make a relational prediction (*e.g.,* nursing notes are referred to less frequently than physicians' notes).

The remaining four hypotheses are testable: all call for some comparison, which means that two variables are involved. The independent and dependent variables for these four hypotheses are as follows:

Hypothesis	**Independent**	**Dependent**
#2	Physician versus other hospital personnel	Frequency of referral to nurisng notes
#3	Location of notes on chart	Frequency of physician referral to nursing notes
#4	Nurses' perception versus actual use	Frequency of referral to nursing notes
#5	Length of patient's stay in hospital	Frequency of referral to nursing notes

Given that the dependent variable is identical for hypotheses two, four, and five, it would be possible to combine these three into one complex hypothesis, although it is not necessary to do so.

Three of the four testable hypotheses (two, four, and five) are directional. They predict some condition under which nursing notes would be more frequently reviewed. Only the third hypothesis is nondirectional—that is, the hypothesis does not predict *where* the nursing notes should be located to increase physicians' use of them. It is not really required that all hypotheses be the same, but unless there is some specific reason not to do so (*e.g.,* inconsistent findings from earlier research relating to only some hypotheses), it makes more sense to state the hypotheses in a consistent format.

D.5. Werronen addressed a research question that is well suited to a qualitative approach—a question about how dyspnea is actually *experienced* by people who have a chronic pulmonary disorder. A quantitative approach could be used to study many aspects of dyspnea (*e.g.,* frequency, intensity, etc.), but only a qualitative approach is well suited to understanding how people *feel* and how they cope with their feelings.

The research problem is one that is of relevance to the nursing profession. By understanding what patients are experiencing, nurses may be better prepared to offer assistance and support. In this instance, the research was also of *personal* interest to the researcher, who was an asthmatic. Many researchers, especially those who conduct qualitative inquiries, select topics in which they have a strong personal investment.

The research questions evolved over the course of Werronen's study. The general research problem was patients' reactions to dyspnea; the initial research question was rather vague—consistent with the limited information that was available on this topic. However, Werronen's research questions became more specific as she collected data and began to see patterns emerging. For example, she noticed that patients with different pulmonary patterns tended to react somewhat differently, and made a decision to explore this in a systematic fashion. Overall, then, Werronen did a good job of selecting an important and interesting topic, addressing it within an appropriate paradigm, and then honing in on some aspects that were manageable within the context of a small-scale and in-depth study.

▧ TEST QUESTIONS AND ANSWERS

Multiple Choice

1. The research question, "What is the decision-making process among intensive care unit nurses who decide to assist terminally ill patients to die?" is:
    - a. Most likely to be addressed using a quantitative approach
    - *b. Most likely to be addressed using a qualitative approach
    - c. Not researchable
    - d. Not appropriately worded

2. The research question, "Should voluntary tubal ligations be performed on women without children?" is:
    - a. Insufficiently significant
    - b. Unfeasible
    - *c. Not researchable
    - d. Acceptable as stated

3. Determining the feasibility of a research question includes all the following considerations *except:*
    - *a. Availability of a relevant theory
    - b. Availability of study participants
    - c. Availability of adequate facilities
    - d. Experience of the researcher

4. The research question, "Does maternal stress during the first trimester of a pregnancy affect the infant's birth weight?" is:

    *a. Acceptable as stated

    b. Not researchable

    c. Not feasible for research inquiry

    d. Not of clinical significance

5. In a research report, the statement of purpose is normally found:

    a. In the abstract

    b. In the first paragraph of the report

    *c. At the end of the introduction

    d. At the beginning of the Method section

6. In a statement of purpose, the researcher often communicates information beyond the problem statement through:

    a. The specification of the population to be studied

    b. The operational definition of the research variables

    c. The prediction of anticipated relationships among variables

    *d. The choice of verbs that suggest the status of knowledge of the topic or the approach to be used in studying the problem

7. A research hypothesis:

    a. Is a set of logically interrelated propositions

    b. Is usually more general in scope than the problem statement.

    *c. Predicts the nature of the relationship between two or more variables

    d. Predicts the absence of a relationship between two or more variables

8. The following are all purposes of the research hypothesis *except:*

    *a. Proving the validity of a theory

    b. Extending human knowledge

    c. Explicating the research question

    d. Providing direction to the research design

9. A research hypothesis indicates the expected relationship between:

    a. The functional and causal nature of the variables

    b. The statement of purpose and the research questions

    *c. The independent variable and the dependent variable

    d. Statistical testing and the null hypothesis

10. Hypotheses are:

    a. Essential to the conduct of respectable scientific enquiry

    b. Needed only when there is an explicit theoretical framework

    *c. Useful in giving direction to quantitative studies

    d. Not appropriate for many nursing research studies

11. The hypothesis, "Women who jog regularly are more likely than those who do not to have amenorrhea" is:
    - a. Null
    - b. Not correctly worded
    - *c. Directional
    - d. Nondirectional

12. A hypothesis that makes an absolute (as opposed to relative) prediction is not:
    - *a. Testable
    - b. Researchable
    - c. Justifiable
    - d. Significant

13. Hypotheses derived from a theory are almost always:
    - a. Null
    - b. Simple
    - c. Complex
    - *d. Directional

14. The hypothesis, "A person's emotional status is not affected by a relocation to a nursing home" is:
    - *a. Null
    - b. Not correctly worded
    - c. Directional
    - d. Nondirectional

15. The hypothesis, "Women who live in rural areas are unlikely to practice breast self-examination" is
    - a. Null
    - *b. Not correctly worded
    - c. Directional
    - d. Nondirectional

16. Which of the following is an example of a complex hypothesis?
    - a. Younger nurses are more likely to hold favorable attitudes toward unionization of nurses than are older nurses
    - b. The greater the amount of reinforcement a new father receives from his wife, the greater the number of functional activities he will perform for the newborn
    - c. Clinical specialist nurses perceive they have more job autonomy in the hospital than do staff nurses
    - *d. None of the above

True/False

(T)   1. A research problem is a situation involving an enigmatic or disturbing situation amenable to disciplined inquiry.

(F)   2. Qualitative researchers begin with a formal research question and then develop hypotheses to be tested while in the field.

(F)   3. The concept of feasibility refers to the potential a problem has for contributing to the nursing literature.

(F)   4. Any question to which an answer is desired is suitable to study by the scientific method.

(T) 5. A research question for a quantitative study contains the major variables in the study and the population being studied.

(T) 6. Criteria for evaluating the value of a research question include its significance to nursing, its researchability, and its interest to the researcher.

(F) 7. All research reports provide a clear purpose statement to guide the reader's understanding of what was studied.

(T) 8. Hypotheses in research reports are typically presented as research hypotheses rather than as null hypotheses.

(F) 9. Hypotheses derived from theory are generally nondirectional in wording.

(F) 10. Hypotheses are more abstract than purpose statements.

(T) 11. Qualitative research almost always proceeds without hypotheses.

(F) 12. Support for a researcher's hypothesis provides proof of the worthiness of the theory from which the hypothesis has been deduced.

(T) 13. A simple hypothesis states the expected relationship between one independent variable and one dependent variable.

(F) 14. Hypotheses must express the expected relationship among at least three variables.

(T) 15. The following is a null hypothesis: "Women who smoke are as likely to have low-birth-weight babies as women who do not."

(T) 16. The following is a directional hypothesis: "The fewer social supports an elderly person has the more likely he or she is to be institutionalized."

Chapter 4
Conceptual Contexts for Research Problems: Literature Reviews and Theoretical Frameworks

◪ STATEMENT OF INTENT

Chapter 4 discusses two important types of intellectual contexts for disciplined inquiries: (1) contexts developed on the basis of a systematic review of existing knowledge via a literature review; and (2) contexts developed within a conceptual or theoretical framework.

The chapter begins by providing assistance to students in locating research reports on a specific topic. The focus is on acquainting students with available bibliographic resources, with an emphasis on electronic database searches. Hands-on exercises in the library are likely to prove helpful here. Chapter 4 also discusses the preparation of literature reviews. This is one of the few chapters in the book in which we provide guidance in actually doing a research activity because both consumers and producers of research prepare written literature reviews. Note, however, that we do *not* have the preparation of a written review as an explicit student objective for this chapter. This is because the chapter teaches some of the mechanics of doing a literature review, but it is premature at this point to expect students to critically evaluate the research literature. This skill should improve as they progress through the remainder of the textbook. We believe, however, that an understanding of what it takes to write a good research review will facilitate students' abilities to critique the literature review sections of research reports.

Chapter 4 also provides some basic information about linkages between theory and research in nursing. The distinction between theories, conceptual models, and frameworks is briefly discussed, as is the distinction between classic theory and descriptive theory. Consumers should be sensitized to the desirability of having a research problem placed in a broad conceptual context because of its potential to enhance the meaningfulness and interpretability of the findings. The chapter makes it clear, however, that most nursing research is *not* conducted within the context of a theoretical framework and that, in many cases, this is perfectly appropriate.

An overview of several specific models/theories used widely in nursing research is provided. Major points to emphasize are that there are alternative ways of explaining and understanding phenomena of interest to nurses and that alternative explanations can be tested in the real world through empirical inquiry. The chapter discusses several different modes in which theory and research are linked (*e.g.,* conducting a study to test a theory, conducting a study to test competing theories, using a theory to explain why certain descriptive findings have been obtained). The text also notes that, unfortunately, some researchers have felt it necessary to invoke a theoretical context that is actually artificial. When a research problem is genuinely linked to a theoretical framework, design decisions, methods of operationalizing variables, data analysis strategies, and interpretations of the findings are driven by that theoretical framework.

▧ COMMENTS ON THE ACTUAL RESEARCH EXAMPLES IN THE TEXTBOOK

Example of a Literature Review from a Quantitative Study

Holditch-Davis and her colleagues (1995) prepared a brief review of the literature on the effects of standardized rest periods on the sleep–wake states of preterm infants as a background for their study on this topic. Here are a few comments about their literature review.

- Their literature review included a great many citations, many of which were for reports published in the 1980s, but also with a good representation of studies from the 1990s. It is, of course, difficult to know if all relevant studies were cited without doing an independent literature search.
- The literature review was well organized, beginning with a documentation of some general needs of critically ill infants, and progressing to a discussion of research on the effects of special interventions that manipulated aspects of the infants' hospital environment. The researchers' literature review supports the need for the study that they undertook.
- The authors adhered to an appropriate style for the literature review presentation. Their assertions are consistently supported by research evidence, and their opinions are not interjected in the review.
- The researchers did an excellent job of critically evaluating the research that had already been done. For example, the authors noted that existing studies have to be interpreted cautiously because of such methodological problems as small sample sizes and poorly matched comparison groups. They also noted that a shortcoming of existing studies is that multiple aspects of the environment were altered simultaneously, making it difficult to determine what modifications led to beneficial effects. Thus, the researchers made a good argument for modifying only a single aspect of the environment, while holding other aspects constant.

Example of a Literature Review from a Qualitative Study

Brodsky (1995) drew on the research literature to frame his research on survivors' perceptions of the psychosocial impact of testicular cancer. Here are a few comments on the literature review in Brodsky's report:

- Consistent with many qualitative studies, the literature review in the introduction was very brief. The two paragraphs are used to (1) document the incidence of testicular cancer in the United States; (2) establish that there have been few studies focusing on testicular cancer patients; and (3) document the increased survival rate in this population. Collectively, this information appears to establish the need for further research, and particularly for in-depth research on a poorly understood group.

- One concern is that all citations in the introduction are for studies that are fairly old; the most recent reference was published in 1984, more than 10 years before Brodsky's study. It is possible that no research was done during the decade before Brodsky's study, but it seems unlikely. If, in fact, there were no studies in the late 1980s and early 1990s, Brodsky might well have pointed this gap out by saying that little work had been done *and* that all work done to date was fairly old and possibly out-of-date.

- Literature is judiciously used in the Discussion section of Brodsky's report as a way of providing even more context for the study findings. Specifically, Brodsky turned to earlier research to determine whether his findings had corroboration. Generally, Brodsky's findings were supported by the findings from other research. Here, too, however, Brodsky relied on corroboration from studies that were fairly old (*i.e.,* mainly studies published in the 1970s and early 1980s).

- The style of the review was generally appropriate, and the organization was generally good. However, Brodsky sometimes relied on quotes from other authors when paraphrasing could easily have been accomplished (*e.g.,* Kennedy's quote).

Research Example of a Conceptual Framework from a Quantitative Study

Pender and colleagues (1990) used the Health Promotion Model (HPM) to study factors that predict employees' adoption of health-promoting lifestyles. Several comments on this study follow.

- This is an excellent example of a study in which the study design and interpretation of the results flow quite naturally from the conceptual framework. There is absolutely nothing contrived about the linkage between the theory and the research in this example.

- The investigators have an obvious commitment to testing the theory, which was developed by the lead author of the research report. Thus, in terms of the issues discussed in the section entitled "Testing and Using a Theory or

Conceptual Framework," this is an example of researchers who moved from a theory to an empirical test of the implications of the theory.

- The report *implies* various hypothesized, causal relationships among the key constructs, based on the HPM. However, it would have been helpful to readers if the investigators had formally specified the hypotheses being tested.

- The researchers' explication of the HPM in the introduction was well placed (within the first few paragraphs of the research report) and sufficiently thorough to give readers an understanding of the model.

- Although this is apparent only in the full research report, each of the constructs described in the textbook and shown in the schematic model (Figure 5-1) was fully and carefully operationalized by the researchers. This illustrates the importance of having the theory–research problem linkage in place *before* undertaking the study. With an after-the-fact linkage, key constructs are rarely operationalized in an optimal way vis-à-vis the theory.

- The findings from the study (which are not summarized in the textbook but may be reviewed in the full report) provide support for the HPM as a method of understanding and predicting health-promoting lifestyles. Further research by this team of investigators and other researchers may continue to confirm the utility of the model or suggest refinements to it.

Research Example of Theory Development from a Qualitative Study

Swanson (1991) developed a descriptive theory of caring based on data from three in-depth qualitative studies. Here are a few comments about Swanson's linkages between theory and research.

- This is a good example of a descriptive theory rather than a classic theory. Swanson's goal was to thoroughly describe the caring process, not to propose relationships between caring and other phenomena.

- Swanson's theory development is greatly enhanced by the fact that she studied caring in three distinct perinatal contexts. As a result, her theory is not restricted to a single situational context. Conversely, she might have further strengthened her position by including contexts other than perinatal ones. Fortunately, her theory is being used as a framework by researchers working with other populations.

- This example shows how theory development progresses. Swanson first identified caring processes in the first study, confirmed and refined them in the second, and added further refinements and elaborations in the third study. By the end of the third study, Swanson was able to provide a conceptual definition of caring that could serve as a foundation for other research (as well as for other applications, such as interventions and curricular developments).

- ■ Consistent with the approach used by qualitative researchers, Swanson offered as evidence for her descriptive theory verbatim excerpts from her study participants. These excerpts greatly enhance the reader's ability to understand the descriptive theory.
- ■ Like all theory, Swanson's theory of caring needs to be corroborated. Swanson's presentation in and of itself offers no way to evaluate the validity of the five-step process.

ANSWERS TO SELECTED STUDY-GUIDE EXERCISES

A.1.

1. c
2. e
3. d
4. e
5. d
6. a
7. b
8. d

A.2.

1. c
2. d
3. f
4. a
5. e
6. b

B.

1. CINAHL
2. Subject
3. Textword
4. Indexes, abstract journals
5. Primary
6. Opinions, anecdotes
7. Findings from other research
8. Relevance
9. Quotes
10. Gaps
11. Critical summary
12. Tentativeness
13. Introduction, discussion
14. Framework
15. Invented (created, constructed)
16. Conceptual models (frameworks, schemes)
17. Words
18. Person, environment, health, nursing
19. Health Promotion Model
20. Borrowed theories

D.3. Forester's literature review has both strengths and weaknesses. It is fairly intelligible, reasonably well organized, and concise. It makes use primarily of research findings (rather than anecdotes or opinion articles), although it seems that more recent research (post-1985) should also have been included. Most of the author's statements are documented, although there are several assertions, particularly in the first two paragraphs, that are not referenced. Also, Forester used primary sources predominately, although there is one instance (in the last paragraph) of a secondary reference that was probably avoidable.

For the most part, Forester used her own words to summarize what is known about PID, but she does use a quote from Eschenbach (in the first paragraph) that is not really justified. Eschenbach's words are not so dramatic, profound, or creative that they cannot be paraphrased. Using quotes in such a situation is only a crutch to avoid abstracting, summarizing, and presenting information in one's own words.

Forester seems relatively unsophisticated with regard to research methods. Her statement in the third paragraph regarding Westrom's "proof" that PID affects fertility suggests that she does not appreciate the limitations of the scientific method. Nowhere in her review does she criticize existing research, describe its limitations, or indicate gaps in what is known.

Forester's summary of existing studies also fails to provide pertinent information in some instances. For example, in the first paragraph, Forester mentions a study by Eschenbach on the incidence of gonococcal infection. The reader would form a different impression of existing knowledge if Eschenbach's study had been based on 50 cases or 5000, yet sample size and sample characteristics are not specified. As another example, Forester describes Westrom's study in detail, yet does not indicate whether the differences between groups were statistically significant.

In summary, Forester's literature review might be considered a good first draft; it is flawed, but improvable. The most serious potential problem is that the review may be inaccurate if more recent research has led to different conclusions about PID. Rewriting this draft will never solve that problem.

D.5. Sterling appears to have started with a theory and then developed the research question based on the theory; the research hypothesis appears to flow directly from the theory. Sterling's process in deriving the research hypothesis might have approximated the following:

- Readings in the general area of social learning theory
- Readings of studies of health-related behaviors as they relate to social learning theory
- Based on these readings, an evaluation of social learning theory as it applies to health-related behaviors
- A deduction that *if* social learning theory were valid, *then* certain predictions could be made about preventive health behaviors
- Finally, the development of the specific research hypothesis

Sterling's findings that people who were more internally oriented were more likely to elect membership in an HMO than externally oriented people could be easily interpreted, given the fact that the hypothesis was developed on the basis of theory. It is not always so easy to interpret one's data, but having a supported hypothesis deduced from theory lends itself to fairly straightforward interpretations. The fact that the hypothesis was supported provides further support to Rotter's theoretical formulations but, of course, does not "prove" its validity. Similarly, if the hypothesis had not been supported, this would not constitute "proof" of the theory's unworthiness, but accumulated instances of research's failure to support a theory would probably seriously undermine its utility.

In the absence of a theory, this particular research problem might never have been studied; the theory indicated a construct in predicting preventive health behaviors (locus of control) that might not have been identified based on casual observations. It should be noted, however, that other conceptual models and theories (*e.g.,* the Health Belief Model, Behavioral Decision Theory) would make similar predictions but might imply a different operationalization of the key constructs.

▧ TEST QUESTIONS AND ANSWERS

Multiple Choice

1. The electronic database most likely to be useful to nurse researchers is:
    *a. CINAHL
    b. CancerLit
    c. Health
    d. MEDLINE

2. In conducting a subject search in an electronic database, you would most likely initiate the search by typing in:
    a. An author's name
    b. Restrictions to the search
    *c. A topic or keyword
    d. A mapping procedure

3. An end-user system:
    a. Is a method of organizing literature review notes
    b. Requires assistance by a librarian
    c. Is the name of an abstracting service
    *d. Allows researchers to conduct their own computer searches

4. In using print indexes, the researcher should ordinarily:
    a. Work forward from the oldest source to the most recent issue
    *b. Work backward from the most recent issue to the oldest source
    c. Search for articles that summarize prior research
    d. Read the accompanying abstract to determine whether the article is pertinent to the topic

5. The type of information in which the researcher is *least* interested when doing a literature review is:
    a. How the variables of interest have been operationally defined in prior studies
    *b. Narrations of a particular author's impression of a given situation
    c. Research results
    d. What research approaches have been used to study similar problems

6. A primary source for a literature review may be defined as:
    *a. A description of an investigation written by the researcher who conducted the study
    b. A summarization of relevant research that has been conducted on the topic of interest
    c. A thesaurus that directs the reader to subject headings germane to the topic
    d. Any retrieval mechanism that helps to locate articles on the area of interest

7. Which of the following journals would most likely contain the highest number of primary sources for a research literature review?

a. *American Journal of Nursing*

b. *Nursing Forum*

c. *Nursing Outlook*

*d. *Western Journal of Nursing Research*

8. Which of the following sentences *best* conforms to the generally acceptable form of a research literature review?

a. It is known that students experience anxiety in taking a test.

*b. Several studies have found that the Lamaze method of childbirth reduces the amount of pain medication required by mothers after delivery.

c. It is clear that motivations cannot be changed overnight.

d. Reinforcement is necessary to maintain positive behaviors.

9. A set of logically interrelated propositions is associated with a:

a. Statistical model

b. Conceptual model

*c. Classic theory

d. All of the above

10. The power of theories lies in their ability to:

a. Capture the complexity of human nature by the richness of the operational definitions associated with the variables

b. Minimize the number of words required to explain phenomena and, thereby, eliminate semantic problems

c. Prove conclusively that relationships exist among the phenomena studied

*d. Specify the nature of the relationships that exist among phenomena

11. The overall purpose of a theory is to:

a. Explain relationships that exist among variables as well as the nature of those relationships

*b. Make scientific findings meaningful and generalizable

c. Stimulate the generation of hypotheses that can be empirically tested

d. Summarize accumulated facts

12. The building blocks for theory are:

a. Propositions

b. Relationships

c. Hypotheses

*d. Concepts

13. The major similarity between theories and conceptual models is that both:

*a. Use concepts as their building blocks

b. Use the deductive reasoning process almost exclusively

c. Contain a set of logically interrelated propositions

d. Provide a mechanism for developing new propositions from the original propositions

14. The Health Promotion Model would best be described as a:
- a. Descriptive theory
- b. Borrowed theory
- c. Grounded theory
- *d. Middle-range theory

15. Which of the following is *not* a central concept in conceptual models of nursing?
- a. Person
- *b. Social support
- c. Health
- d. Environment

16. The nurse-theorist Orem developed the:
- a. Conservation Model
- b. Health Promotion Model
- c. Adaptation Model
- *d. Model of Self-Care

True/False

(T) 1. A textword search allows searchers to look for topics in text fields of records in the electronic database.

(F) 2. The CINAHL electronic database covers all published nursing studies back to the early 1900s.

(T) 3. Abstract journals summarize articles that have appeared in other journals.

(F) 4. A published literature review article would be considered a primary source for a person doing a literature review on the same topic.

(F) 5. Information from anecdotal and opinion articles is usually included in a research literature review.

(F) 6. A well-written literature review is characterized by numerous quotations from research studies.

(F) 7. Paraphrasing, rather than directly quoting from an article, is a common flaw in literature reviews.

(F) 8. A good literature review includes the researcher's opinions on the issues being investigated.

(T) 9. The literature review section should conclude with a critical evaluation of knowledge on the problem of interest.

(F) 10. "Research has proved that cigarette smoking causes lung cancer" is an appropriately worded statement for a literature review.

(T) 11. Classic theories explain not only the relationships between variables but also the nature of those relationships.

(T) 12. Descriptive theories involve a thorough description or classification of a single phenomenon.

(F) 13. Through research replications, theories can be definitively proved.

(T)   14. Failure of research to disconfirm a theory increases support for the theory.

(F)   15. Research endeavors that are not based on theory have little, if any, scientific use.

(F)   16. Grounded theory is to descriptive theory as a schematic model is to a conceptual framework.

(T)   17. Schematic models attempt to represent reality with a minimal use of words.

(F)   18. A conceptual model may be defined as a well-formulated deductive system of abstract formal propositions.

(T)   19. All studies have a framework, even though not all studies are based on a theory or conceptual model.

(T)   20. Mishel's Uncertainty in Illness Theory is an example of a middle-range theory.

Chapter 5
The Ethical Context of Nursing Research

◨ STATEMENT OF INTENT

The purpose of Chapter 5 is to familiarize students with the basic principles involved in the protection of the rights of human subjects in research. Humans are the study participants in most nursing studies, and it is important for consumers to be sensitive to the major ethical principles governing the conduct of nurse researchers. It is also important, however, to understand that the need to adhere to ethical guidelines sometimes conflicts with the basic aim of conducting rigorous research. Therefore, instructors need to help students develop an appreciation for various ethical dilemmas in which competing demands on the researcher must be balanced. An important concept in this regard is the risk/benefit ratio. Because many nurse researchers study vulnerable groups, students need to develop special sensitivity in evaluating the ethical aspects of studies in which vulnerable subjects were used.

◨ COMMENTS ON THE ACTUAL RESEARCH EXAMPLES IN THE TEXTBOOK

Research Example From a Quantitative Study

Some comments regarding the ethical aspects of Holdcraft and Williamson's (1991) study are presented here.

- The risks in this study could be described as minimal. Although it is possible that completion of the Miller Hope Scale might be somewhat stressful for a few subjects, it is unlikely to be more stressful than other aspects of the patients' experiences or treatment. The risk/benefit ratio seems acceptable.
- Informed consent was obtained from each subject; however, given the fact that these were vulnerable subjects, it is not clear that each subject was capable of giving fully informed, voluntary consent. The report does not indicate any exclusion criteria—circumstances under which the severity of the illness might have caused a subject not to be asked to participate. Although this does not necessarily mean that the researchers did *not* exclude sub-

jects who were incapable of giving informed consent, there is simply inadequate information in the report to know for sure. There is no mention of any discussion with legal guardians.

- The questionnaires were returned by the patients in a sealed envelope, which protected their privacy. However, given that the subjects completed the questionnaires twice, anonymity could not have been assured. That is, the researchers had to be able to match the two sets of questionnaires for subjects, and they therefore used a system of identification numbers to link the pretreatment and posttreatment questionnaires. Because of their inability to have the questionnaires completed anonymously, however, the researchers took extreme precautions to safeguard the patients' confidentiality. Moreover, the investigators explicitly noted that all identifying information was destroyed at the end of the study.

Research Example From a Qualitative Study

Some comments regarding the ethical aspects of the qualitative study by Kearney et al. (1995) are presented here.

- This study posed a number of ethical challenges, because of both the content of the interviews and the characteristics of the study participants. The researchers generally dealt with ethical issues in a thoughtful and compassionate manner.
- The researchers undertook several steps to protect the study participants from harm. The interviewers gave the informants considerable leeway in controlling how much information was divulged. They also made referrals to appropriate service agencies for women in need of help. The study participants may also have found the interview itself somewhat therapeutic.
- Participation in the study was presumably voluntary, and all women signed informed consent forms. However, participants were recruited through health and social service agencies, and some women may have believed that they had no choice but to volunteer. It is also possible that the $40 stipend was sufficiently generous as to make it difficult for some women to decline participation. Another issue is the informants' ability to truly understand what they were agreeing to do. However, it is likely that these concerns were reviewed and appropriately addressed by the two IRBs that reviewed the study protocols.
- The researchers took great pains to protect the privacy of their informants. The women in the study decided where the interview would take place. They were also asked to use pseudonyms—thereby ensuring that the interviews had an element of anonymity. Additionally, the researchers obtained a Certificate of Confidentiality from the National Institute of Drug Abuse, which made it impossible for participants who divulged criminal actions to be criminally prosecuted.

◩ ANSWERS TO SELECTED STUDY-GUIDE EXERCISES

A.1.

1. d		7. b	
2. b		8. a	
3. c		9. c	
4. b		10. a	
5. a		11. b	
6. d		12. d	

B.

1. Dilemmas	6. Self-determination
2. Nuremberg code	7. Full disclosure
3. *Belmont Report*	8. Anonymity
4. Harm	9. Vulnerable
5. Minimal risks	10. Institutional Review Boards

D.2. Portnoy's study presents some potential problems from an ethical point of view. The most fundamental problem is that the study participants were not really given an opportunity to give their informed consent, and the intent of the researcher was not fully disclosed to subjects before their volunteering to participate. Indeed, the researcher deliberately deceived the study participants regarding the purpose of the study. The researcher's rationale was that deception was necessary to observe the subjects' "natural" handling of an emergency situation. If the students had been told that the study concerned their reactions in a crisis, their behavior would probably not have been spontaneous, and the results would probably have been meaningless. In other words, if informed consent had been obtained, the study might not have been worth doing.

Some people might argue that it would have been preferable simply to *observe* student nurses' reactions in a setting in which crises might occur so that deception would not be necessary. There are three difficulties with such an approach, however. First, the incidence of crises in such a setting might be relatively low, so that a great deal of time would be needed to observe 100 such situations. Second, not all crises are the same; in a natural setting, the researcher would lose control over the stimulus designed to elicit the student nurses' behaviors. Finally, in a natural setting, the behaviors of others would contaminate the subjects' behaviors. Students might be relatively passive knowing that more experienced personnel were available.

In the current situation, therefore, the use of deception might be justified. Although the students probably did not derive much personal benefit from their participation (except the receipt of a $10 subject stipend), neither is it likely that they suffered any physical or psychological harm. It appears as though they were treated equitably, their privacy was protected, and the researcher demonstrated courtesy to participants by promptly debriefing them at the end of the study. Moreover, the results of the study might be of considerable importance in curricular improvements for nursing students or in helping nurse administrators to make effective staffing decisions. On balance, the risk/benefit ratio seems acceptable.

Portnoy could be more confident that her research was ethically acceptable by conducting a small preliminary study (*e.g.,* with 10 or so students). She could then question these subjects afterward and ask about their reactions to the deception and method of data collection. She could also ask them whether they would have been willing to participate even with full knowledge of what the research entailed. Portnoy should, in any event, be careful to have all aspects of the research reviewed by an appropriate human subjects committee or Institutional Review Board.

▨ TEST QUESTIONS AND ANSWERS

Multiple Choice

1. The Tuskegee Syphilis Study violated which of the following ethical principles?
   a. Freedom from harm
   b. Right to self-determination
   c. Right to fair treatment
   *d. All of the above

2. The regulations affecting the ethical conduct of research sponsored by the federal government were incorporated into:
   a. The Nuremberg Code
   b. The Declaration of Helsinki
   *c. *The Belmont Report*
   d. The Code of Ethics of the American Psychological Association

3. Debriefing sessions are:
   a. Discussions with prospective subjects before a study to obtain informed consent
   *b. Discussions with subjects after a study to explain various aspects of the study and provide a forum for questioning
   c. Discussions with a human subjects committee before a study to obtain permission to proceed
   d. None of the above

4. All the following are potential benefits from participating in a study *except*:
   a. Monetary gains
   b. Access to a new and potentially beneficial treatment
   c. Opportunity to discuss personal feelings and experiences with an objective listener
   *d. Opportunity to run a debriefing session

5. The three primary ethical principles described in this chapter include all of the following *except*:

    a. Beneficence

    b. Respect for human dignity

    *c. Informed consent

    d. Justice

6. If a researcher unobtrusively studies interactions among patients in a psychiatric hospital, which ethical principle may be violated?

    a. Confidentiality

    b. Freedom from harm

    *c. Right to self-determination

    d. All of the above

7. The safeguard mechanism by which *even* the researcher cannot link the participant with the information provided is called:

    a. Confidentiality

    *b. Anonymity

    c. Informed consent

    d. Right to privacy

8. Confidentiality of subjects can be increased by:

    *a. Avoiding the collection of any identifying information

    b. Avoiding introducing the subjects to any of the research personnel

    c. Placing all identifying information on computer files rather than manual files

    d. All of the above

9. Vulnerable subjects would include:

    a. Women hospitalized for a mastectomy

    b. Members of a senior citizens group

    c. People with a speech impediment

    *d. Pediatric clients

10. Informed consent is not obtained when:

    a. The researcher pays the subjects a stipend

    *b. The researcher collects information covertly

    c. The risk/benefit ratio is low

    d. The researcher's study is determined to be exempt from IRB review

11. In a qualitative study that involves multiple contacts between the researcher and study participants, the researcher may negotiate a(n):

    a. Informed consent

    b. Stipend

    *c. Process consent

    d. Risk/benefit ratio

12. In research reports, researchers are most likely to discuss which of the following aspects of their study:

    *a. Whether informed consent was obtained

    b. Whether the subjects were vulnerable

    c. What the risk/benefit ratio was

    d. Whether the subjects were debriefed at the end of the study

True/False

(F)   1. There is never any justification for violating the three primary ethical principles articulated in the Belmont Report.

(F)   2. The last major transgression of ethical principles in the conduct of research occurred in the experiments conducted by the Nazis.

(T)   3. Ethical dilemmas are inevitable in the conduct of scientific research.

(T)   4. Minimal risks are ones that are no greater than those a person normally confronts in daily life.

(T)   5. The principle of self-determination concerns whether participation in a study was coerced.

(F)   6. Freedom from harm and the right to privacy are the two principles on which informed consent is based.

(F)   7. Guaranteeing confidentiality to study participants means that the researcher could never link the data gathered to the person who supplied the data.

(T)   8. Observations through a one-way mirror may undermine a subject's right to full disclosure.

(T)   9. From a research standpoint, a person who does not have the competence to give his or her informed consent is considered a vulnerable subject.

(F)   10. An Institutional Review Board reviews the scientific merits of completed research.

Designs for Nursing Research

PART III

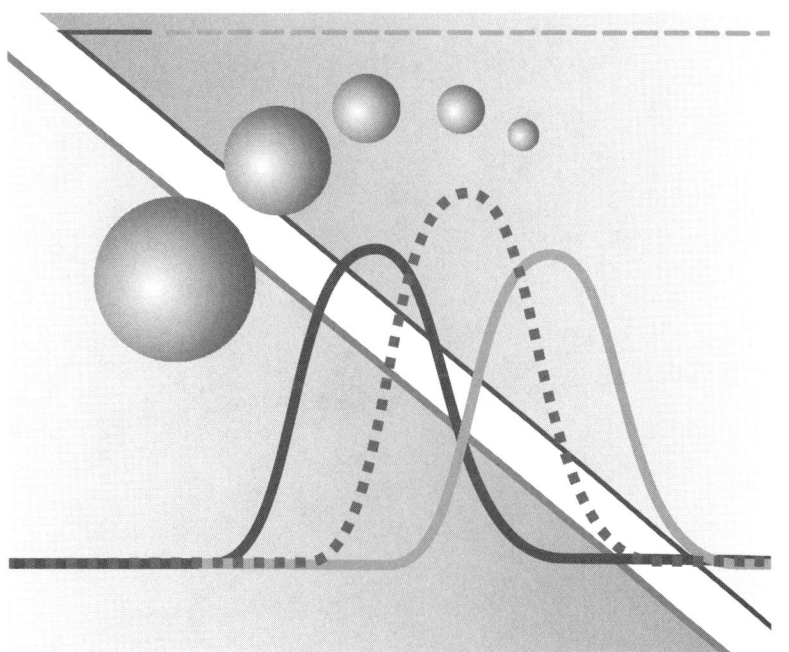

Chapter 6
Research Design for Quantitative Studies

▧ STATEMENT OF INTENT

Chapter 6 is one of the most important chapters of the textbook because it introduces consumers to principles that are critical to evaluating the basic architecture of a quantitative study. The chapter is devoted to a discussion of various dimensions of research design and techniques of research control.

The first section provides students with an overview of some of the fundamental features of research design in quantitative studies. The major dimensions of research design (*e.g.,* whether there is an intervention; whether the study is cross-sectional or longitudinal) are described. An important lesson here is that researchers generally have considerable flexibility in designing studies, but design decisions have implications for the interpretability of the study findings.

The next few sections of the chapter explain differences between research designs in which the researcher does or does not introduce an intervention or treatment—the differences between experimental, quasi-experimental, and nonexperimental research. These sections introduce students to several important research design issues, such as randomization and manipulation. The relationship between research design and causal inferences is underscored. The text points out, however, that although nonexperimental research (and even quasi-experimental research) limits the researcher's ability to draw conclusions about causality, many research problems are simply not amenable to an experimental design.

The chapter also explains how studies can be designed to maximize the quality and interpretability of the results. An especially important section discusses methods of building controls into the design of a research study. Means of achieving control over extraneous variables that are both extrinsic to the research situation and intrinsic to the research subjects are discussed. This discussion is especially important because consumers must consider what design alternatives might have strengthened a study and how believable are the findings of a study, given the limitations of the design. Chapter 6 also introduces the important concepts of internal and external validity and points out that compromise is often needed to balance design requirements for these two criteria.

COMMENTS ON THE ACTUAL RESEARCH EXAMPLES IN THE TEXTBOOK

Example 1: Research Example of a Longitudinal Experimental Evaluation

Koniak-Griffin, Ludington-Hoe, and Verzemnieks (1995) undertook an interesting experimental study. Below are some selected comments about the study, with particular emphasis on its design features.

- The study was a true experiment. There was manipulation of the independent variable (type of stimulation), a control group, and subjects were randomly assigned to conditions. The design could be described as an after-only (or posttest only) design, because measures of the dependent variable (mental and psychomotor development) were not collected before any intervention. However, it was an after-only design with multiple "after" points of data collection. The study is therefore longitudinal (a follow-up study) and can be considered an evaluation because it evaluated the impacts of an experimental intervention.

- The design seems highly appropriate. By using a true experimental design with random assignment, the authors were able to draw conclusions about the effects of the interventions without having to worry if the infants in the four groups were developmentally different at the outset. (Furthermore, the researchers can be commended for comparing the background characteristics of subjects in the research groups; their similarity at the outset gives some indication that the random assignment was successful in equalizing the groups.) It might also be noted that an after-only experimental design was a reasonable choice. For example, a repeated measures design could not have been used because the outcomes of interest were measured months after the intervention.

- The periods of follow-up were scheduled for 4, 8, and 24 months after birth of the child. These follow-up points appear to be appropriate given the researchers' interest in charting the child's development.

- Attrition was a problem in this study, as it is in most longitudinal studies: about two out of five of the original subjects (39%) did not participate in the 24-month follow-up. The researchers indicated that those who dropped out of the study were generally similar to those who remained in the study with respect to background characteristics and dependent variables at the 4-month point. However, there was one significant difference, and so departure from the study was not totally random. It is commendable that the researchers examined possible attrition biases. Nevertheless, it is possible that the internal validity of the study was somewhat compromised. (The report indicates that there were differences between attriters and non-attriters with regard to 4-month developmental scores, but it does not indicate whether treatment groups were differentially affected by attrition.)

■ The researchers controlled various external factors by collecting all of the follow-up data in a single type of setting, namely, in the study participants' homes. Further control was introduced by having the data collected by nurses who were not aware of the participants' treatment group.

Example 2: Research Example of a Quasi-Experimental Study

Pickler and her colleagues (1993) used a strong quasi-experimental design to study the effect of nonnutritive sucking (the independent variable) on bottle-feeding stress in preterm infants. Here are some selected comments regarding the design of this study:

■ This study is not experimental because the infants were not randomly assigned to the two groups. (Unfortunately, the authors did not indicate why an experimental design was ruled out; presumably there were practical constraints that made randomization unfeasible.)

■ Although infants were not randomly assigned to the two groups, the design is nevertheless a strong one—essentially it is a time series nonequivalent control group design. Data were collected at multiple points (including before and after the nonnutritive sucking) from both the experimental group and the comparison group.

■ In addition to the fact that the researchers included a comparison group of infants, they took extra care to ensure the comparability of the two groups by matching the infants in terms of important characteristics: their gestational age, birth weight, gender, and race. (Unfortunately, there is no information regarding how the matching was performed—*e.g.,* within what ranges birth weights were matched, as an indication of the precision of the matching. The absence of significant differences on these matching variables is not totally reassuring because of the very small sample size.)

■ Despite the absence of details about the matching, the design is sufficiently strong that the results are unlikely to be biased by extraneous variables— although we cannot rule out the possibility that extraneous variables other than those used for matching purposes were differentially distributed in the two groups and influenced the observed differences in the behavioral state. Definitive conclusions are, moreover, premature because of the small sample size and the many nonsignificant results.

Example 3: Research Example of a Nonexperimental Survey

Pollow and her colleagues (1994) conducted an excellent survey that has important implications for health-care workers. Some comments regarding the design and conduct of this survey are as follows:

■ This study is an example of a large-scale survey that yielded an extensive amount of information from a large sample of subjects. It is clear that a great deal of time and care (and resources) were devoted to the planning and execution of this survey. Because the study relied on an excellent sampling strategy (probability sampling) and had a large sample, the study's findings are likely to be robust and generalizable. Although the response rate (79%) was less than ideal, this rate compares quite favorably with rates typically achieved with elderly subjects.

- Commendably, the data were collected by personal interviews rather than by questionnaire or telephone. Such a strategy is especially important in studies of the elderly, whose rates of volunteering for studies is usually low. Moreover, telephone surveys would probably have been inappropriate for many elderly people (*e.g.,* those with hearing impairments) and would not have reached the elderly who do not have telephones.
- A very important benefit of personal interviews in this particular study was that the interviewers were able to actually examine the bottles or boxes of medications that the elderly respondents were using. This possibility undoubtedly greatly enhanced the accuracy of the data.

▧ ANSWERS TO SELECTED STUDY-GUIDE EXERCISES

A.1.

1. b		6. a	
2. b		7. d	
3. a		8. a	
4. d		9. b, c	
5. b		10. d	

A.2.

1. a, d		5. d	
2. c		6. b	
3. a		7. a	
4. b		8. b	

B.

1. Experimental, nonexperimental
2. Comparison
3. Independent
4. Treatment (intervention)
5. Systematic bias
6. Pretest
7. Factorial design
8. Levels
9. Double blind
10. Repeated measures
11. Causality (cause-and-effect relationships)
12. Comparison
13. Preexperimental
14. Time series
15. Equivalent (equal)
16. Nonexperimental
17. Independent
18. Causal (cause and effect)
19. Retrospective

20. Longitudinal
21. Follow-up studies
22. Surveys
23. Evaluation
24. Key informant
25. Methods

26. Constancy
27. Generalizability
28. Internal
29. Mortality
30. Maturation

C.2.

a. Cannot
b. Can
c. Can
d. Cannot
e. Cannot
f. Cannot
g. Can
h. Cannot

i. Can
j. Can
k. Cannot
l. Can
m. Can
n. Cannot
o. Can

C.5.

4.a. Nonexperimental
4.b. Nonexperimental
4.c. Both
4.d. Both
4.e. Nonexperimental

5.a. Nonexperimental
5.b. Both
5.c. Nonexperimental
5.d. Both
5.e. Nonexperimental

D.2. DeSeve used a time series (quasi-experimental) design to test her hypothesis that the relaxation and biofeedback intervention had an effect on women's menopausal symptoms. Although the design has some limitations, DeSeve's collection of data over an extended period provided some measure of protection against instability or misleading findings that might arise with data collected at only two times (before and after).

One of the problems with this design is that, although there are many data collection points, they are compressed in time. If this 5-week period is unusual or atypical in any respect, or if something external to the study is happening concurrent with the intervention, the results could be biased or distorted.

Another difficulty with the design is that there are *too many* data collection points. From a practical point of view, consider the problems involved in analyzing these data. From a methodologic point of view, the multiple measurements could result in inaccurate data. For example, some subjects might get bored with the task of recording their symptoms and might not pay much attention to the information they are providing. Others might be influenced in what they report on one day by what they reported on the previous day.

Because of these concerns, a more reasonable design might be recommended. For example, one design would involve eight data collection points: on 4 consecutive weeks before the intervention and on 4 consecutive weeks after the intervention. The subjects might be instructed to record symptoms each Wednesday, for example, except during the 3-week intervention. The elimination of data collection during the treatment period might help prevent or minimize the Hawthorne effect, that is, biases resulting from the subject's awareness of being part of a study.

The best design, of course, would be an experiment wherein a randomized group of women did *not* get the new intervention. Random assignment might have proved unfeasible for DeSeve, but she probably could have obtained a nonrandomized comparison group. When nonequivalent control group and time series designs are combined, the resulting design is fairly powerful.

D.4. Auclair's study is inherently nonexperimental. Her independent variable, social and emotional supports, cannot, as defined, be manipulated by the investigator unless some serious ethical transgressions are committed (*e.g.*, prevention or enforcement of interaction between subjects and their kin or friends). It might, of course, be possible to design an intervention with the aim of adding to the subjects' social support networks; the effectiveness of this intervention could then be tested with an experimental design. However, this would be a different study.

The study as described is prospective in nature. Auclair first ascertained the subjects' degree of social supports. Then, 6 months later, she collected information on the subjects' mental and physical health. The use of a prospective design is commendable; such a design permits the researcher to establish the sequence of events. Auclair, however, did not capitalize on this aspect of her prospective design. We cannot really be sure that the group with low social support did not have initial health problems that could have *led* to the disengagement from or rejection by friends and kin. Auclair would have done better to collect data on her dependent variables at both data collection points and then analyze the relationship between social supports and *changes* to the measures of health and morale. This would at least have enabled her to ascertain that the subjects' social support status preceded their health status.

Even with this modification, however, there are problems in using correlational data to test cause-and-effect relationships. Three conditions are necessary to establish causality. The first, determining the existence of an empirical association, has been accomplished in this example. The second, determining that the cause preceded the effect, could be established with the changes suggested above. The third condition, however, concerns ruling out the possibility that the underlying causal mechanism is not some third factor that is correlated with both the independent variables and dependent variables. In experiments, this condition is satisfied because groups are (presumably) equivalent with regard to everything except exposure to the independent variable. In ex post facto research, many extraneous variables can confound the results if they are not controlled. In the current example, the underlying cause of the subjects' health status might be their personalities: outgoing and trusting people may be more motivated to maintain a strong social support system *and* obtain adequate health care. Other extraneous variables that could be responsible for the observed relationship between social supports and health could be marital status, age, economic circumstances, and urban versus rural residence, to name only a few.

D.6. Neudel used a nonexperimental, retrospective design to study the relationship between the use of an intrauterine device (IUD) and the incidence of pelvic inflammatory disease (PID). The question she was asking is one that can best be addressed with an experimental design—whether the use of an IUD *causes* PID. It would not be feasible, however, to randomly assign subjects to different contraceptive user groups. Ethical constraints prohibit the use of an experimental design.

Neudel did a number of things to help increase both the internal and external validity of her study. In terms of internal validity, she used the matching procedure to control for two variables: the woman's age and her marital status. By controlling such variables, she presumably controlled for the likelihood that the woman would be in need of regular, effective contraception. She might also have controlled for parity as well. Other variables that might have been considered include socioeconomic status (which would provide a rough control for health status) or some other, more direct measure of the woman's health or health care use. The problem, however, is that the researcher would have had difficulty in matching on more than two or three variables. (However, she could also have used another method of control, such as homogeneity; for example, she could have limited her study to married women or to women with at least one child.) Furthermore, because the design was retrospective, she was limited to controlling variables that could be obtained from information available in the patients' records.

The use of a retrospective design poses numerous other problems. One issue, for example, is the question of whether the retrospective data are accurate. Neudel looked at records going back 2 years to determine whether the women had had IUDs inserted during that period. However, what if the IUD had been inserted in another facility? There is no way of knowing whether such circumstances might be more prevalent in the PID or non-PID group, and therefore there is no way of knowing whether there are systematic biases. Neudel attempted to compensate for this problem in part by trying to locate the women for whom the records were incomplete; however, she probably was unable to always tell when the records were incomplete. Furthermore, contacting the women could potentially result in biases stemming from, for example, recall problems or the researcher's inability to find all the subjects.

Another problem that emerges in retrospective research is whether the samples are truly representative. In a prospective design, the researcher would begin with a large sample of women—some of whom are or would be users of the IUD and others who would not. Then these women would be followed over time to determine who would eventually contract PID. Beginning with a group that already has PID makes it impossible to have the sample include women who might have PID but do not have it diagnosed or treated. This might result in a systematic bias in the sample with regard to such factors as social class or health beliefs.

It is commendable that Neudel did try to ensure that the sample was varied at least with regard to social class by drawing on patients from four different types of health facilities. This feature enhances the external validity of the study. Because the women were, for the most part, unaware of their subject status, many of the threats to the external validity of this study (such as the Hawthorne effect or novelty effects) are not relevant.

The researcher's conclusion that the use of an IUD was a causative factor in the development of PID was unwarranted, given the limitations of this research. The researcher was able to demonstrate that a relationship between the two variables existed, but other criteria for demonstrating causality could not be established. That is, Neudel could not demonstrate that the temporal sequencing was as hypothesized (perhaps in the PID group, the PID was already present at the time of insertion of the IUD). But, more important, the design failed to control for a number of extraneous variables. Perhaps the IUDs were more likely to be inserted in multiparous women, and parity rather than IUD insertion is the causative factor. Perhaps PID is more common among women with numerous sexual partners or among women who smoke heavily, a condition that might preclude the use of oral contraceptives. In short, the investigator used a design that makes it difficult to rule out competing explanations for the results.

D.8. Poole used a cross-sectional design to study changes over time in a person's intellectual and motor capacity. In selecting such a design, Poole had to assume that the 70-year-olds tested at the time of the study would have scored similarly to the 30-year-olds had the 70-year-olds been tested 40 years earlier. This assumption is probably not warranted. Within two generations, many social changes have occurred that could affect test scores. For example, many of those in the older group might have been born outside the United States and might not be native English speakers. This might artificially depress test scores, regardless of true intelligence. The older generation is also less "test-wise" (*i.e.*, not as familiar with the mechanics of taking paper-and-pencil tests) and might be less motivated than younger subjects to complete or try to do well on a speeded test.

The results could also be biased in the other direction (*i.e.*, the results might underestimate the "deteriorating" effect of aging). For example, if intelligent people can earn more money and live longer than less intelligent people because of better nutrition and health care, then those in the sample of 70-year-olds might overrepresent healthy, intelligent people. Poole realized this possibility and partially controlled for it by adding social class as a kind of blocking factor. This precautionary measure is commendable. A tighter control over social class might have strengthened the design even further. For example, the blocking variable could have included three or four levels of income or could have been defined as number of years of education.

Social class and gender were the only extraneous variable that Poole attempted to control. The internal validity of the study could have been improved by the control of other selection factors that could have biased the findings. Several possible extraneous variables include place of birth (United States versus another country); childhood area of residence (urban versus rural); and ethnicity. These could be controlled statistically by matching, by being built into the design, or by narrowing the definition of the population.

Even with additional controls, Poole's cross-sectional design could still contain many sources of bias. The above measures would be most successful in addressing the threat of selection bias but would not address the threats of history or mortality. The most useful design for Poole's research question is a longitudinal study, in which the same subjects would be tested at different ages to see whether their intelligence and motor capacity declined with age. Needless to say, such an enterprise would require considerable resources and patience and many years to complete. Even such a study would be exposed to several validity threats. For example, differential mortality might introduce bias (*e.g.,* if poorer people tended to die at an earlier age).

In summary, Poole has posed a research question for which there is no infallible design. The question is inherently nonexperimental (one cannot manipulate the subjects' ages), making causality difficult to establish. A longitudinal design would have been preferable to a cross-sectional design; however, tighter controls would have reduced the principal problem in the existing design: the threat of selection biases. It is precisely in research problems such as this one that the need for replication and alternative research strategies are critical.

◪ TEST QUESTIONS AND ANSWERS

Multiple Choice

1. The research design for a quantitative study involves decisions with regard to all of the following *except*:
     *a. Whether there will be a theoretical context
     b. Whether there will be an intervention
     c. What types of comparisons will be used
     d. How many times data will be collected

2. One of the functions of a rigorous research design in a quantitative study is to have control over:
     a. Dependent variables
     b. Independent variables
     c. Blocking variables
     *d. Extraneous variables

3. A true experiment requires all the following *except*:
     a. Control
     b. Manipulation
     *c. Double-blind procedures
     d. Randomization

4. When the researcher simultaneously manipulates two independent variables, the design is a:
     a. Pretest–posttest design
     *b. Factorial design
     c. Time series design
     d. Randomized block design

5. How many hypotheses can be tested in a two-factor design?
     a. 1
     b. 2
     *c. 3
     d. 4

6. The use of a table of random numbers for randomly assigning subjects to groups reduces the possibility of a:

*a. Selection threat

b. History threat

c. Mortality threat

d. Maturation threat

7. Which of the following must be present in quasi-experimental research?

a. A comparison group

*b. Manipulation of a variable

c. Matching of subjects

d. Randomization

8. A one-group, pretest–posttest design is an example of a:

a. Time series design

b. True experimental design

c. Quasi-experimental design

*d. Preexperimental design

9. For a researcher to examine interaction effects, which of the following designs must be used?

a. A pretest–posttest design

b. A case-control design

*c. A factorial design

d. A times series design

10. In a nonequivalent control group design, the most serious threat to internal validity is:

a. Testing

*b. Selection

c. Maturation

d. Mortality

11. What feature of a nonequivalent control group design makes it quasi-experimental rather than pre-experimental?

a. Manipulation of the independent variable

b. Lack of randomization

*c. The use of a pretest

d. The use of a posttest

12. Which of the following research designs does *not* necessarily involve collection of pretest data?

a. Nonequivalent control group design

b. Time series design

c. Before–after design

*d. Repeated measures design

13. A study is internally valid if:

*a. All alternative explanations of results can be ruled out

b. An experimental design was used

c. Randomization was used

d. A causal relationship is detected

14. One weakness associated with ex post facto research is the:

a. Artificiality of the setting in which it occurs

b. Difficulty in linking the research to a theoretical framework

*c. Problem of self-selection into groups

d. Inability to generalize the findings beyond the sample

15. Which of the following research designs is *weakest* in terms of the researcher's ability to establish causality?

    a. Experimental
    c. Prospective
    *b. Retrospective
    d. Quasi-experimental

16. In an ex post facto study, compared with an experimental study, the researcher forfeits control of:

    *a. The independent variables
    c. The criterion variables
    b. The dependent variables
    d. The attribute variables

17. In a study in which medical diagnosis is the independent variable, an ex post facto study is essential because the independent variable:

    *a. Is inherently not manipulable
    c. Is practically not manipulable
    b. Is ethically not manipulable
    d. All of the above

18. A study that followed, over a 20-year period, users and nonusers of oral contraceptives to determine if there were any long-term side effects would be called a:

    a. Time series
    *c. Prospective study
    b. Retrospective study
    d. Repeated measures study

19. Research projects that collect data at one time are referred to as:

    a. Retrospective studies
    c. Longitudinal studies
    *b. Cross-sectional studies
    d. Panel studies

20. Which of the following designs involves the use of the same subjects at several points in time?

    a. Trend study
    *c. Panel study
    b. Cross-sectional study
    d. All of the above

21. The US Census is an example of:

    *a. A survey
    c. A needs assessment
    b. An evaluation
    d. An experiment

22. If a researcher wanted to determine how well a prenatal program was meeting its objectives, the type of research would be:

    a. A case-control study
    c. A needs assessment
    *b. Evaluation research
    d. Survey research

23. Which of the following approaches could use an experimental or quasi-experimental design?

    a. Meta-analysis
    c. Survey
    b. Needs assessment
    *d. Evaluation

24. Suppose a nurse researcher is interested in learning whether a self-administered health history questionnaire yields results comparable to a personal-interview health history form. The research approach to such a study would be:

    a. Meta-analysis
    *c. Methodologic
    b. Evaluation
    d. Survey

25. Needs assessments often involve the use of:
- a. Cost-benefit analyses
- b. Meta-analyses
- *c. Key informants
- d. Extraneous variables

26. Using the principle of homogeneity to control for extraneous variables has implications for:
- a. Interaction effects
- *b. Generalizability of the findings
- c. Precision of the effects
- d. Bias in the design

27. Ways in which a researcher can control extraneous variables that are intrinsic to the subjects include:
- a. Using a homogeneous sample
- b. Analysis of covariance
- c. Matching subjects
- *d. All of the above

28. The most effective method of controlling extraneous variables is by:
- a. Analysis of covariance
- b. Matching
- *c. Randomization
- d. Blocking

29. The researcher must know in *advance* the extraneous variables that are to be controlled for which of the following procedures?
- a. Matching
- b. Blocking
- c. Analysis of covariance
- *d. All of the above

30. When subjects' behaviors are affected not by the treatment per se but by their knowledge of participating in a study, the generalizability of the results are limited because of the influence of the:
- a. Experimental effect
- *b. Hawthorne effect
- c. History effect
- d. Novelty effect

True/False

(T) 1. The researcher manipulates the independent variable in both experimental and quasi-experimental research.

(F) 2. The experimental treatment is the dependent variable.

(F) 3. Quasi-experimental research requires the use of a comparison group.

(F) 4. The most effective method for equalizing groups in a study is matching.

(T) 5. The time series design is a type of quasi-experimental design.

(F) 6. The type of research that has the most controls associated with it is called quasi-experimental.

(T) 7. The pretest–posttest design collects data from subjects twice.

(F) 8. Clinical trials generally use a time series design.

(T)   9. Preexperimental, quasi-experimental, and experimental research have one common feature: manipulation.

(T) 10. The purpose of both experimental and ex post facto research is to determine the relationships that exist between the variables of interest.

(T) 11. The researcher does *not* manipulate the independent variable in ex post facto studies.

(F) 12. A researcher would choose a quasi-experimental approach when ethical constraints prevent manipulation of the independent variable.

(T) 13. Prospective nonexperimental studies move from presumed causes to presumed effects.

(F) 14. Retrospective designs are stronger in determining causal relationships than are prospective designs.

(T) 15. Prospective designs are inherently longitudinal.

(F) 16. A study that focused on development among preterm infants would ideally use a cross-sectional design.

(T) 17. A survey researcher collects information about the status quo of a situation.

(F) 18. One of the limitations of survey research is that the approach lends itself only to the collection of objective facts.

(F) 19. A needs assessment provides decision makers with information on the success or worth of a program.

(F) 20. Evaluation research requires a nonexperimental research approach.

(F) 21. Randomized block designs involve the simultaneous manipulation of two or more independent variables.

(T) 22. The use of a homogeneous sample helps to control the influence of extraneous variables in a study.

(T) 23. A blocking variable refers to a nonmanipulated independent variable that is built into the study.

(T) 24. The threat of mortality refers to differential attrition from groups.

(F) 25. The major threat to the internal validity of a nonexperimental study is maturation.

Chapter 7
Qualitative Research Design and Approaches

◈ STATEMENT OF INTENT

The purpose of Chapter 7 is to acquaint students with some features of research design for qualitative studies. Research design elements for qualitative studies often evolve in the field, but nevertheless several aspects of quantitative design are also of relevance in qualitative design, such as *where* the study should take place, and *how often* data should be collected. In qualitative studies, however, descriptions of the research design are often after-the-fact characterizations of what emerged in response to ongoing data collection and analysis rather than specifications of preplanned activities.

Chapter 7 also provides a brief summary of the research traditions that have guided qualitative inquiry—traditions that have provided a foundation for numerous nursing studies. Each research tradition focuses on certain types of research question—and each has its own approach to the collection and analysis of qualitative data. Only three research traditions—ethnography, grounded theory, and phenomenology—are elaborated on, because these are the three traditions that have proved of most interest to nurse researchers.

The search for truth and meaning is at the heart of scientific inquiry, and new approaches for discovering them are constantly evolving. An emerging trend in nursing research, as well as in other disciplines, is the use of multimethod research, in which qualitative and quantitative data are integrated. This chapter is designed to alert students to the many ways in which integration can advance nursing science. The fundamental rationale for blending different approaches is that integration improves the validity and interpretability of a study. The chapter describes several specific strategies for productively combining qualitative and quantitative analyses and also reviews some of the barriers—which are eroding over time—to integration.

COMMENTS ON THE ACTUAL RESEARCH EXAMPLES IN THE TEXTBOOK

Example of an Ethnographic Study

Dreher and Hayes undertook an interesting and complex field study within the ethnographic tradition. Some selected comments about the design and conduct of their study follow:

- The researchers ensured that they would thoroughly understand the context of the use of ganja among Jamaican women by spending a very long time in the field—6 years. Through such intensive, long-term study, the researchers could be relatively sure that they had been able to gain an emic perspective on the phenomena under investigation. Furthermore, by remaining in the field for 6 years, they were actually in a position to observe changing trends in the use of ganja among women.

- The researchers gathered a wealth of data that likely increased the validity of their findings. For the qualitative portion of their study, they interviewed many women and actively participated in their lives. They got to know not only all of their study participants but the whole community in which they lived.

- A very interesting feature of this research is that it combined an ethnographic study with a clinical study. Not only did the data from the two parts of the study supplement each other nicely—the work in the ethnographic study helped to form the basis for the clinical study: through their in-depth knowledge of the culture, the researchers were better able to adapt the child assessment instruments and administer them properly.

Example of an Integrated Study

Reed (1991) investigated the mental health of a group of the oldest-old in relation to a developmental resource referred to as self-transcendence. Below are several comments relating to the researcher's data.

- The researcher elected to use both qualitative and quantitative data in her study. Given the nature of the research problem, this integration seems appropriate. The investigator's dependent variable (mental health status) is one that has been rigorously studied and for which many psychometrically sound quantitative measures exist. For example, the Center for Epidemiological Studies Depression Scale (CES-D) is a widely used measure of mental health in nonclinical populations.* Conversely, the construct of self-transcendence has had little research attention, and therefore, in-depth

---

*See the fictitious study and critique by Bristol in the Study Guide for an example of using the CES-D.

questioning in this area seems highly desirable to more fully comprehend its dimensions and boundaries.

- The researcher was unusually thorough in describing her methods of analyzing the qualitative data. Her article included a chart outlining the seven iterative steps undertaken to move from transcribed interviews to the entries in her two-dimensional matrix.
- Reed's qualitative analysis was systematic and methodical and yielded four major clusters within the self-transcendence construct. Her table (reproduced in the textbook as Table 7-3) provided an excellent mechanism for displaying the clusters, the categories within the clusters, and actual samples of data illustrating the meaning of the categories.
- The qualitative data allowed the researcher to more fully understand, describe, and illustrate the construct of central interest in her research: self-transcendence. Moreover, the qualitative data were juxtaposed with depression scores to maximize the potential of the qualitative data to illuminate the relationship between self-transcendence and mental health status.
- Although the researcher was careful in explaining the steps taken in the data analysis, supplementary efforts she may have undertaken to validate her thematic categorization were not described. For example, the author does not indicate that a second person was asked to code a portion of the qualitative material to evaluate intercoder reliability. Nor does the report indicate that the categorization was shared with respondents to determine whether the thematic analysis made sense to those whose experiences and feelings were being studied.
- Regrettably, the report does not provide much specific information regarding the extent to which the qualitative analysis supported the validity of the structured and Self-Transcendence Scale (STS), perhaps because the researcher intends to focus on this issue in a separate research report. Although the report does not specifically discuss the issue of content validity of the STS, we may infer that some exists because the correlational analysis between the STS and CES-D was substantiated by the matrix analysis in which CES-D scores were juxtaposed with the qualitative categories.

Example of a Phenomenologic Study

Coward's (1995) study used Reed's framework as a starting point for her phenomenologic study. Here are a few comments about that study:

- Coward's focus, consistent with a phenomenologic orientation, was on the *lived experience* of self-transcendence among women with AIDS. The women in the sample were asked to fully describe their thoughts, feelings, and perceptions with regard to any experience of self-transcendence that had occurred since being diagnosed with AIDS.

- This study was somewhat unusual in that it was based on a previously developed framework. However, neither is this study unique: a number of phenomenologic nursing studies do indicate linkages with other theorists, often with Rosemary Parse.
- The main source of data in this study came from in-depth interviews with a small sample of women, as is usually the case with a phenomenologic inquiry. (Actually, 10 is a rather large sample for such a study.)
- The study did not describe the actual steps and procedures (*i.e.,* bracketing, intuiting, and so forth). However, this is consistent with the fact that most qualitative research reports do not provide this level of detail. Moreover, not all phenomenologic studies involve these steps, so perhaps this one did not.
- Coward's research report was greatly enriched by the selection of excellent excerpts that highlighted the experiential themes that emerged in the analysis.

◪ ANSWERS TO SELECTED STUDY-GUIDE EXERCISES

A.1.

1. b	6. a
2. a	7. b
3. d	8. c
4. c	9. d
5. b	10. c

A.2.

1. c	5. c
2. a	6. a
3. c	7. c
4. d	8. a

B.

1. Anthropology, psychology, sociology	5. Spatiality, corporeality, temporality, relationality
2. Cultures	6. Grounded theory
3. Researcher as instrument	7. Complementary
4. Essence	8. Validity

C.2.

a. Grounded theory	c. Discourse analysis
b. Ethnography	d. Phenomenology

D.2. Clark's main approach was quantitative—the collection of structured data by means of a survey; however, she embedded a qualitative data collection approach (unstructured interviews) within the survey. By combining strategies that yielded both qualitative and quantitative data, Clark was able to gather a rich set of data. The structured interviews allowed her to collect specific information about breast-feeding practices and duration and about specific predictors of breastfeeding, such as demographic characteristics and personal attitudes. The structured interviews also allowed her to measure a number of psychological variables using established scales whose psychometric properties were known in advance. Using sophisticated statistical procedures, these data would allow her to explain and predict variation in breastfeeding status and duration, but these analyses might not really allow her to *understand* this variation. For example, if the statistical results indicated that teenage mothers who did not breastfeed their babies had lower self-esteem than those who did, what does this really *mean*? *How* does low self-esteem function to inhibit breastfeeding? It is possible that the in-depth data, collected by means of an unstructured topic guide, would shed light on the meaning of the findings. It is also possible that the qualitative analyses would confirm that, in this hypothetical example, self-esteem is an important construct in teenagers' decision making relating to breastfeeding. It therefore seems likely that the collection of both qualitative and quantitative data in Clark's study enhanced the validity and interpretability of the findings.

Nevertheless, it is also possible to imagine ways in which the study design and data collection effort could be further strengthened. First, it might be pointed out that Clark's decision to conduct in-depth interviews with only those teenagers who were interviewed at home was ill advised. It is true that such in-depth interviews are not appropriate for the telephone and should have been conducted in a face-to-face situation. However, in Clark's study, all of the in-person interviews were conducted with teenagers who could not be interviewed by telephone (presumably because the teenagers did not have telephones or had such irregular hours that they could not be contacted by telephone), thereby leading to a situation in which all of the in-depth interviews were conducted with an unusual subset of the sample. Clark should have made arrangements to conduct some in-depth interviews with telephone respondents.

Clark's study would probably also have been strengthened if the data had been collected at multiple times. For example, she might profitably have begun with some in-depth interviews to better understand the nature of the breastfeeding decision. If she had done so, she might have opted for different scales and questions to be included in the structured interview. For example, the in-depth interviews might have shown the importance of such constructs as body image or cognitive maturity—constructs that were not measured in the structured interviews at all. As another alternative, it might have been useful to postpone the in-depth interviews until after the quantitative data had been analyzed. To pursue the example suggested above, if the statistical analysis of the data from the structured interview had indicated that self-esteem was important in understanding breastfeeding patterns, then perhaps a large portion of the in-depth interviews could have focused on this construct. An iterative approach to multimethod research offers many advantages.

▨ TEST QUESTIONS AND ANSWERS

Multiple Choice

1. All of the following are issues that a qualitative researcher attends to in planning a study *except*:
    - a. Selecting a site
    - b. Determining how best to gain entree in key settings
    - *c. Selecting research instruments
    - d. Determining the maximum amount of time available for field work

2. Which of the following design features can apply to both a qualitative and quantitative study?
    - a. Manipulation of the independent variable
    - *b. Cross-sectional or longitudinal data collection
    - c. Control over extraneous variables
    - d. Random assignment of study participants

3. The research tradition known as *ethnoscience* has its roots in the discipline of:
    - *a. Anthropology
    - b. Philosophy
    - c. Psychology
    - d. Sociology

4. The research tradition known as *ethnomethodology* has its roots in the discipline of:
    - a. Anthropology
    - b. Philosophy
    - c. Psychology
    - *d. Sociology

5. The research tradition known as *hermeneutics* is closely allied to another research tradition known as:
    - a. Ethnography
    - *b. Phenomenology
    - c. Ethology
    - d. Symbolic Interaction

6. Ethnographers strive to:
    - *a. Understand human cultures
    - b. Develop an etic perspective
    - c. Link the etic and emic perspectives into a unified whole
    - d. All of the above

7. Which of the following is *not* a step in the phenomenologic approach?
    - a. Bracketing
    - *b. Inferring
    - c. Analyzing
    - d. Describing

8. A researcher gets on an elevator and, instead of facing forward, faces backward toward other elevator passengers. This would be an example of:

a. An ethnographer's attempt to gain an emic perspective

b. A phenomenologist's effort to appreciate the essence of what the passengers are experiencing

*c. An ethnomethodologist's attempt to understand the social expectations regarding elevator riding

d. A discourse analyst's attempt to listen to people's conversation on an elevator

9. Which of the following approaches involves the use of a procedure known as constant comparison?

*a. Grounded theory

b. Ethnography

c. Phenomenology

d. Ethology

10. The integration of qualitative and quantitative analyses in a study or cluster of studies serves the important purpose of:

a. Providing researchers with different skills an opportunity to collaborate

*b. Enhancing the validity of the study

c. Allowing research subjects to select whether they prefer an unstructured or structured method of responding

d. Enhancing the likelihood that the study will be published

True/False

(F) 1. Design decisions evolve while the study is in progress in both qualitative and quantitative studies.

(F) 2. Unlike quantitative researchers, qualitative researchers do not use group comparisons to promote understanding of phenomena of interest.

(T) 3. Qualitative researchers eschew the concept of constancy of conditions.

(T) 4. A qualitative researcher typically enters the field not knowing what is not known.

(F) 5. Human ethology studies the essence of human behavior through in-depth discussions with study participants.

(F) 6. Phenomenologists focus on the manner by which people make sense of social interactions.

(F) 7. Bracketing refers to the process of separating qualitative data from quantitative data.

(T) 8. Constant comparison is a technique used in grounded theory in developing theoretical categories.

(F)   9. Qualitative data are more profitably integrated into studies that are basically quantitative than vice versa.

(T)   10. The validity of a study is enhanced when a hypothesis is supported by complementary types of data.

Chapter 8
Sampling Designs

▨ STATEMENT OF INTENT

Chapter 8 introduces students to the concept of sample selection for both quantitative and qualitative studies. As in other aspects of study design, sampling issues are handled quite differently by researchers working within different paradigms in terms of goals, approaches, and criteria for evaluating adequacy from the larger population in which a researcher is interested.

With regard to quantitative research, the chapter describes several types of nonprobability and probability samples and offers guidelines for assessing the quality of the researcher's sampling approach. Detailed procedures concerning the complex topic of sample size are not discussed, but the point is emphasized that sample sizes in quantitative studies should generally be large, especially if the population is heterogeneous with respect to the variables of interest. The principles underlying a power analysis are also described, and an example is used to show that generally fairly large samples are needed to adequately test research hypotheses. The point is made, however, that size alone cannot guarantee a good sample. A sample for a quantitative study is good if it is *representative,* and several factors—most importantly, size, method of selection, response rate, and subject attrition—determine a high-quality sample. The issues of representativeness of a sample and the adequacy of sample sizes are particularly important because many quantitative nursing research studies have weak sampling designs.

Qualitative researchers employ very different strategies, and are guided by different considerations than quantitative researchers. The chapter describes several alternative approaches that are used to enhance the *information-richness* of the data obtained in a qualitative study. In a qualitative study, random selection is not only not attempted, it is eschewed. Sample size is also guided by data adequacy rather than by the need to achieve certain statistical goals.

▨ COMMENTS ON THE ACTUAL RESEARCH EXAMPLES IN THE TEXTBOOK

Research Example of a Quantitative Study

Ferrans and Powers's (1992) sampling design has numerous commendable features as well as a few shortcomings. Below are a few comments regarding their research sample.

- The investigators used a highly sophisticated sampling plan that provided an excellent opportunity to achieve a representative sample. All adult, in-unit hemodialysis patients in most counties in Illinois had an opportunity (an *equal* opportunity) of being selected for inclusion in the sample. Such a sampling plan is considerably more rigorous than that used in most nursing studies.

- The accessible population consisted of adult in-unit dialysis patients in 93% of the counties in Illinois. Unfortunately, the report did not indicate why 7% of the counties were excluded, nor *which* 7% were excluded. For example, the exclusion of Cook County—where Chicago is located—would certainly result in a sample not totally representative of Illinois. It is also not clear what the overall target population was without knowing whether Cook County was included. Quality of life might well be affected by urban versus rural residence, for example. The report also does not explain why patients undergoing treatment in Veterans Administration (VA) hospitals were excluded, nor ways in which such patients might be expected to be different from those treated in non-VA hospitals.

- Of the sampled patients who could have completed a questionnaire, 57% actually responded, which is a reasonably good response rate for data collected by questionnaire. Many completed questionnaires had to be discarded, however, because of missing information, so that the actual response rate was 46%.

- The final sample consisted of 349 subjects, a sample size that is considerably larger than in most nursing studies. Inasmuch as the focus of the study was not on the testing of research hypotheses (*e.g.,* comparing dialysis patients with cancer patients in terms of quality of life), this sample size was probably adequate.

- One excellent feature of this study was that the investigators directly examined the representativeness of the sample, vis-à-vis the accessible population, with respect to basic demographic information. They learned that the sample and the accessible population were comparable in terms of a number of important characteristics that might be expected to affect a person's perceptions of their life quality (*e.g.,* gender and length of time on dialysis). Significant differences were found on two variables (race and age); however, these characteristics are likely to be highly related to quality-of-life perceptions. Thus, the investigators discovered some bias in their sample. This discovery makes it possible for consumers to better interpret the results of the study.

- Despite some evidence of bias, the investigators had an extremely strong design. Given the methodologic nature of the study, it seems unlikely that the results were strongly affected by the bias. That is, the overall soundness of the QLI would not likely have been judged much differently if a more representative sample had been obtained. But, of course, this possibility does exist. Replication of the study with older and nonwhite patients would be desirable.

Research Example of a Qualitative Study

Quinn's (1993) sampling plan was geared to the needs of her qualitative research, as discussed below.

- Quinn's approach to sampling is a good example of the sampling decisions that a qualitative researcher makes. She began by simply defining the eligibility criteria for inclusion in the sample and then recruiting nurses who met those criteria.
- As Quinn collected and analyzed her in-depth data, she was better able to identify data needs, and so her sampling decisions were then guided by theoretical sampling considerations. In other words, her sampling requirements emerged on the basis of the data, not on the basis of a preconceived notion of what her needs would be.
- This example clearly shows an advantage to a flexible approach. Had the sampling plan been designed in advance, Quinn might not have realized the importance of including nurses from different shifts.
- Quinn's sampling can be described as theoretical sampling because decisions were based on the researcher's need to select participants on the basis of information needs emerging in the early findings. Although Quinn's approach cannot really be described as a maximum variation sampling approach, nevertheless it appears that her overall aim was to include nurses with a broad range of perspectives.
- Quinn's sample size (20 nurses) was undoubtedly adequate to achieve data saturation, although the report did not explicitly say so.

▨ ANSWERS TO SELECTED STUDY-GUIDE EXERCISES

A.1.

1. b	6. c
2. c	7. a
3. a	8. a
4. b	9. d
5. b	10. b

A.2.

1. c	6. b
2. a	7. c
3. d	8. d
4. b	9. a
5. c	10. d

B.

1. Sample	10. Multistage
2. Representativeness	11. Sampling interval
3. Biased	12. Sampling error
4. Homogeneous	13. Accessible
5. Accidental sample	14. Increases
6. Strata	15. 30
7. Judgmental; purposeful; theoretical	16. Information
8. Simple random sampling	17. Homogeneous; maximum variation
9. Weighting	18. Typical case

C.2.

a. Multistage (cluster)	e. Quota
b. Convenience (accidental)	f. Extreme (deviant) case
c. Simple random	g. Snowball (network)
d. Systematic	

C.3. Sampling interval = 22; elements = 134, 156, 178

D.2. Dresser's sampling design can best be described as quota sampling. She had the names of students from three types of nursing programs and used essentially convenience sampling to fill 100 slots for each type. (Schools themselves were selected according to a quota system, with two schools per type.) Dresser's sampling design has some good features. In particular, her selection of 100 students from the three programs guaranteed that all three types would be adequately represented in the survey. Her procedure was thus better than it would have been had she merely obtained the lists and then surveyed the first 300 students she could locate.

Dresser's method of obtaining respondents for each of her three cells, however, exposed her to a considerable risk of bias. Given that local telephone directories were used to locate subjects, it is highly probable that certain students were automatically excluded from the sample. Students who had moved from the area, had unlisted telephone numbers, had changed their surnames, or had telephones listed under roommates' names had no opportunity to be included in the study. Such students probably differed systematically from students who were accessible through telephone directories. For example, students who had moved from the area might consist of a disproportionately high percentage who got good job offers, who got no job offers, or who decided to go to graduate school. There is no way of knowing the nature and extent of the biases in Dresser's sample.

Several steps could be taken to improve Dresser's design. She would probably have had better success in locating graduates had she sought the cooperation of either the nursing schools or the state licensing agency. Another alternative would have been to contact students before graduation and obtain their addresses or the names and addresses of people through whom they could be contacted, such as parents or siblings. If these steps had been taken, Dresser might have been able to select a random sample of graduates.

If Dresser could not follow the above suggestions for some reason, she still could have introduced somewhat more control into her design. For example, she could have selected a random sample of 100 students from each program type and then made a more concerted effort to locate the selected graduates. She could have asked for leads or contact information from the students she *was* able to locate, or she could have inaugurated a postal search by mailing a letter to prospective participants at the school of nursing.

Even modest adjustments might well have improved the representativeness of the final sample. It would probably have been relatively easy to introduce additional strata into the sampling design. Then, even with convenience sampling within strata, according to a quota system, some biases might have been eliminated or reduced. Examples of other strata about which information could have been obtained from either the nursing school or prospective respondents include gender, field of specialization, and whether the subject was an honors student.

The abstract did not specify Dresser's target and accessible populations. It is probably safe to assume that her accessible population was recent nursing graduates residing in the Washington, DC, area. The most conservative definition would be that the accessible population consisted of graduates of six Washington-area nursing schools residing in or near Washington, with a published telephone number. It would take a giant leap of faith to assume that these 300 subjects adequately represent the target population of recent nursing graduates in the United States, as implied.

Dresser's sample size is modest for a survey of this type because one would expect considerable diversity (heterogeneity) with respect to job-seeking experiences. Still, 300 is a fairly respectable number and is probably adequate for descriptive purposes. If Dresser had taken steps to improve the representativeness of the subjects, her sampling approach would have been acceptable.

One final consideration involves Dresser's stratification. Her plan involved the use of disproportionate sampling (*i.e.,* 100 may be a 10% sample of baccalaureate students from the two schools but a 30% sample of diploma students from the two diploma schools). Given the probability that Dresser's sample is not representative of the target or accessible populations, it is somewhat irrelevant whether proportionate or disproportionate sampling was used. If she had been able to obtain a stratified random sample through a method such as that described earlier, a proportionate sampling design would probably have been the best way of obtaining accurate estimates of population values.

D.4. Downie began with two purposive samples of couples who had fertility impairments—those who had and those who had not (yet) achieved a pregnancy. Within each group, Downie sought to maximize variation with regard to several aspects of the fertility problem and its treatment.

By using a maximum variation approach, Downie was able to get a handle on the breadth of issues that related to these couples' quality of life. Based on what she learned from the initial five or six interviews, Downie then sought couples whose experiences had the most potential to achieve data saturation on the themes that had emerged. Had Downie planned her sampling strategy in advance, she might have missed some opportunities to enrich her data in theoretically important ways.

It is unclear from the brief summary whether the total sample size of 20 couples was adequate. However, because sampling decisions were guided by the desire for data saturation, one must assume that the researcher was successful in achieving it.

◪ TEST QUESTIONS AND ANSWERS

Multiple Choice

1. Sampling may be defined as the:

  a. Identification of the set of elements used for selecting subjects

  *b. Process of selecting a subset of the population to represent the entire population

  c. Aggregation of subjects who meet a designated set of criteria for inclusion in the study

  d. Technique used to ensure that every element in the population has an equal chance of being included in the study

2. Bias in a sample for a quantitative study refers to:

  a. Lack of heterogeneity in the population on the attribute of interest

  b. Sample selection in nonprobability-type sampling

  c. The margin of error in the data obtained from samples

  *d. Systematic overrepresentation or underrepresentation on the attribute of interest vis-à-vis the population

3. Strata are incorporated into the design of which of the following types of samples:

  a. Systematic

  b. Purposive

  *c. Quota

  d. Simple random

4. The methods of nonprobability sampling include all the following *except*:

  a. Convenience

  *b. Cluster

  c. Purposive

  d. Quota

5. Of the following, the type of sampling design that would be especially likely to yield a representative sample is:

  *a. Systematic

  b. Convenience

  c. Purposive

  d. Quota

6. Of the following types of sample, which one is considered to be the weakest for quantitative studies?
   *a. Convenience
   b. Quota
   c. Purposive
   d. Systematic

7. The type of nonprobability design that is most likely to yield a representative sample is:
   a. Convenience sampling
   b. Purposive sampling
   *c. Quota sampling
   d. Network sampling

8. The procedure of weighting is associated with which type of sampling design?
   a. Proportionate sampling
   *b. Disproportionate sampling
   c. Simple random sampling
   d. Quota sampling

9. A researcher used a probability-type systematic sampling plan. The sample size was 200. The sampling interval was 250. The first element drawn was 196. The second element would be:
   a. 396
   b. 450
   *c. 446
   d. 646

10. A researcher used a systematic sampling design. The known population size is 3200, and the desired sample size is 160. What is the sampling interval?
    a. 16
    *b. 20
    c. 160
    d. 320

11. Which of the following terms does not belong with the others?
    a. Purposeful sample
    b. Purposive sample
    c. Theoretical sample
    *d. Volunteer sample

12. A sampling strategy that is diametrically opposed to maximum variation sampling is:
    a. Extreme case sampling
    *b. Homogeneous sampling
    c. Intensity sampling
    d. Typical case sampling

True/False

(F) 1. Sampling bias would be of greater concern in studying body temperatures in healthy adults than in studying their attitudes toward abortion.

(T) 2. The major criterion in assessing the adequacy of a sample in a quantitative study is the degree to which it represents the characteristics of interest in the population.

(T) 3. Random selection is used in all types of probability sampling designs.

(F) 4. If a probability sampling design has been used, the researcher can safely generalize to the target population.

(F)   5. Systematic sampling involves the successive random sampling of units from largest to smallest.

(T)   6. In a quantitative study, larger samples are more likely to represent the population on the attribute of interest than smaller samples.

(F)   7. Snowball sampling is to convenience sampling what cluster sampling is to simple random sampling.

(F)   8. Each element in the population has an equal chance of being selected in a nonprobability-type sampling plan.

(T)   9. Systematic sampling may be of a probability or nonprobability nature.

(F)   10. The researcher hand-picks people to be included in a study in quota sampling.

(F)   11. Differences between population values and sample values are referred to as weighting errors.

(T)   12. Power analysis is used to estimate the sample size needed to adequately test research hypotheses.

(F)   13. A major criterion for assessing the adequacy of a sample in a qualitative study is the degree to which a theory has been developed to adequately describe the population.

(T)   14. In a qualitative study, sample size decisions are often guided by the principle of data saturation.

(F)   15. The sampling strategy that involves the selection of extreme cases is referred to as intensity sampling.

Collection of Research Data

PART IV

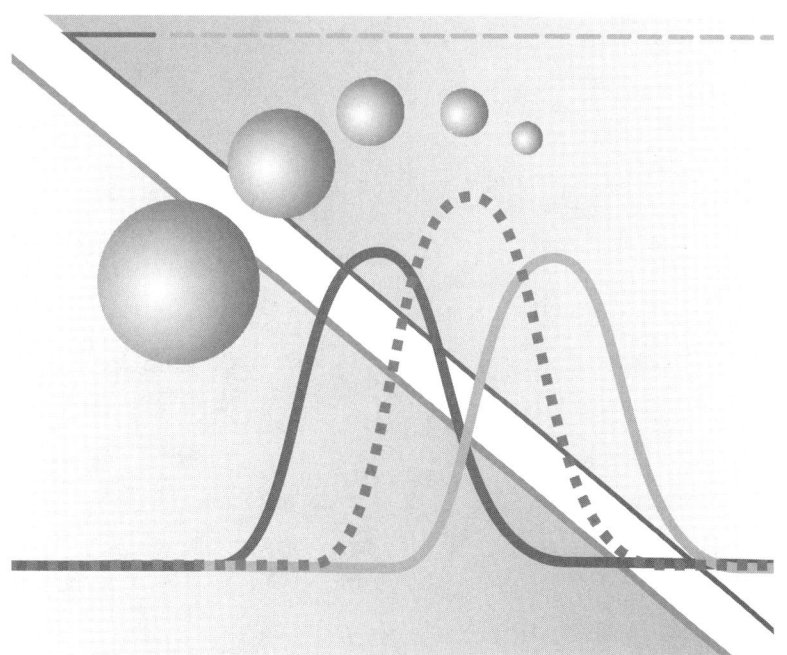

Chapter 9
Methods of Data Collection

◩ STATEMENT OF INTENT

Chapter 9 describes the major alternative methods of obtaining research data. After an introductory section that discusses the use of existing data versus the gathering of new data, the text goes on to explain that methods of gathering data differ on four critical dimensions (structure, quantifiability, researcher obtrusiveness, and objectivity) and in basic approaches (self-report, etc.). It is important for consumers to understand how much flexibility a researcher has in operationalizing variables and to realize that the decisions that the researcher makes are open to critical scrutiny.

The chapter then describes the major features of the primary forms of data collection used by nurse researchers, namely, self-reports, observational techniques, and biophysiologic measures. Both structured forms of data collection amenable to quantitative analysis and unstructured forms of data collection amenable to qualitative analysis are described.

The section on self-reports discusses various forms of unstructured self-report techniques, such as focused interviews, life histories, and focus group interviews. With respect to more structured self-report techniques, the chapter presents some basic information on the use of questionnaires and interview schedules. The differences between these two forms of structured self-reports are described in some detail, with the intent of providing readers with an understanding of the situations in which one or the other techniques might be appropriate. The chapter also presents some basic concepts in the construction and interpretation of composite self-report scales, which combine multiple measures to form a single score of a particular attribute—typically a social–psychological attribute such as attitudes. Other less widely used forms of self-report (vignettes, Q sorts, and projective techniques) are briefly described. Finally, the strengths and limitations of self-report techniques (including response set biases) are discussed. Consumers should recognize the problems of self-report techniques as well as situations in which they are appropriate.

The next section of Chapter 9 introduces readers to procedures used to collect data by direct observation. Observational methods are often especially useful to nurse researchers because many patient outcomes are amenable to observation. Both structured and unstructured observations are described and evaluated. General principles for constructing checklists and rating scales are also presented. Finally, the issue of observational biases is discussed, and criteria for critiquing observational methods are presented.

Biophysiologic measures are discussed next. These measures have assumed greater significance to nurse researchers in the past two decades because of the growing emphasis on clinical research. Therefore, it is important for consumers to understand their applications, strengths, and limitations.

Guidelines for the critical evaluation of the various data collection approaches are presented within each major section. Separate guidelines are also presented to help consumers evaluate the procedures used to collect research data.

▨ COMMENTS ON THE ACTUAL RESEARCH EXAMPLES IN THE TEXTBOOK

Example 1: Scales and Biophysiologic Measures

Topf (1992) undertook a well-designed experimental study in which the independent variable—noise level and instruction regarding control over noise—was manipulated. The dependent variables were measured using structured self-reports (including scales) and biophysiologic instrumentation. Here are a few comments on the researcher's data collection plan.

- The biophysiologic instrumentation constituted an excellent means of gathering detailed, sensitive, and accurate information regarding the sleep patterns of the subjects. Clearly, the data on actual sleeping behavior could not have been measured through self-report. Sleeping behavior could have been measured through direct observation, but observation would likely have been less accurate. Moreover, many of the variables measured (*e.g.*, time spent in different periods of sleep) are *not* amenable to observation.
- The researcher took considerable care in converting biophysiologic information into usable quantitative data. A doctorally prepared polysomnographer scored the sleep records. A second doctorally prepared polysomnograph technician reviewed a sample of the records, and the results of the two scorers were compared. Agreement between the two was high.
- The researcher's decision to obtain a subjective measure of sleep was possibly unnecessary, given the excellent objective measures of sleep available (moreover, the subjective measure was not really used in any of the analyses). Conversely, this measure was easily obtained and possibly has methodologic value in that the measure correlated as high as .50 with one of the biophysiologic measures.
- The scale used to measure stress due to hospital noise seemed like an excellent choice. The tape-recorded noises were carefully controlled, which ensured that each subject would be reacting to the same stimulus. There

were enough items on the scale to derive a stable estimate of how stressed different people were by hospital noises.

- The administration of the social desirability scale is often a useful means of determining bias in self-reports. It is not clear, however, that this scale was needed in this study. Although the study did include several self-report measures, the variables under study were not ones that were likely to inspire a need among the subjects to distort responses to look good.

- The high degree of structure of the data collection measures seems appropriate, given the nature of the research question. However, a few open-ended questions regarding the subjects' experience in the sleep laboratory or about their regular sleeping patterns and reactions to noise might have enriched the study.

Example 2: Participant Observation and Unstructured Self-Report

Chase (1995) conducted an in-depth ethnographic study of critical care units. Here are some comments on Chase's methods of data collection.

- Chase nicely integrated several types of data collection methods. Chase's methods varied in terms of basic approach (self-report and observation); focus (from general and nonspecific to more focused); setting (both an open heart surgical ICU and a general surgical ICU); and type of study participants (nurses and physicians).

- Chase used data collection methods that were well suited to her desire to describe the social context for clinical judgments in a critical care environment. She obtained information about the activities, patterns, and processes within the ICU directly through observation, and she obtained information about perceptions and clinical judgments through her interviews.

- The degree of structure in Chase's study was totally consistent with the purpose of the study. It is difficult to imagine, for example, how the use of an observational checklist or rating scale would have yielded an understanding of the overall social context of the ICU. Moreover, this study exemplifies one of the advantages of a flexible data collection plan. The researcher began with making general observations about the dynamics within the ICU and noticed that an important aspect of what was going on concerned communication patterns. Subsequent observations then focused on those patterns. The researcher also decided, on the basis of her early field work, that gathering data at another site would enhance her ability to interpret her data.

- A noteworthy aspect of Chase's study is that she spent 2 years in the field collecting her data. It is through such long, intensive field work that an ethnography can be successful in understanding a cultural context.

Example 3: Structured Interview, Scales, and Records

Yates and Belknap (1991) also used multiple methods of data collection—all of them structured—in their study of the factors predictive of physical functioning after a cardiac event. The following comments relate to issues in their data collection plan.

- Given the researchers' interest in identifying predictors of physical functioning, the use of highly structured and quantifiable measures seems appropriate.
- The psychosocial variables in this study (depression, mastery, and self-esteem) were appropriately measured with widely used, standardized scales. (The report provides a good description of each scale, including information about quality.)
- The use of visual analog scales (VASs) to measure various aspects of the subjects' recovery and subjective feelings of physical recovery seems appropriate. VASs yield highly sensitive measures and are relatively easy for subjects to complete. (It might be noted, however, that these VASs were specifically developed for this particular study, but there is no information on whether they were adequately pretested. This, of course, does not mean that they were not.)
- A highly objective and sensitive measure of physical functioning was obtained by means of the symptom-limited exercise test (SXT). (To ensure accuracy of scoring, the researchers had two scorers independently score the tests; agreement was nearly perfect.) Additional physical measures were obtained from hospital records.
- Data from the interviews and the SXT were collected, on average, within less than a week of one another, thereby minimizing any possibility of distortions stemming from the data being collected at different points in the subjects' recovery. (Additionally, the researchers analyzed the extent to which length of time between the two sets of measurements or whether having the SXT or interview first affected any of the results.)

▧ ANSWERS TO SELECTED STUDY-GUIDE EXERCISES

A.1.

1. b		5. d	
2. a		6. a	
3. c		7. b	
4. c		8. c	

A.2.

1. c	6. b
2. b	7. b
3. a	8. a
4. a	9. c
5. a	10. a

B.

1. Existing data
2. Historical research
3. Secondary analysis
4. Structure, quantifiability, researcher obtrusiveness, objectivity
5. Topic guide
6. Focus group interview
7. Closed-ended (fixed-alternative)
8. Open-ended
9. Pretest
10. Closed-ended (fixed alternative)
11. Scale
12. Declarative
13. Reversed
14. Bipolar adjectives
15. Extreme response set
16. Response set biases
17. Vignettes
18. Behavior
19. Reactivity
20. Participant observation
21. Single, multiple, mobile
22. Logs, field notes
23. Category system
24. In vivo
25. In vitro

C.3.

$Y = 11; Z = 26$

C.4.

A = Acquiescence   C = Extreme response set
B = None   D = Nay-sayers' bias

C.5.

a. 5	f. 1
b. 1	g. 5
c. 1	h. 5
d. 5	i. 5
e. 5	j. 1

Minimum score = 10, maximum score = 50

D.2. Alongi used a questionnaire in her study of adolescent drug use patterns, an efficient method of collecting data from a large sample of respondents who were geographically dispersed in 25 different communities. The time and expense required to interview 3568 students would have been extremely high. There are other advantages to the use of questionnaires in this particular study. Given that the investigation concerned drug-use habits, a questionnaire that gave total anonymity probably enhanced the truthfulness of student responses. It is easier to admit to socially unacceptable behavior when one believes that no one will be able to learn your identity.

One of the chief disadvantages of questionnaires is that response rates tend to be low, resulting in the possibility of a biased sample. Alongi's method of distribution probably resulted in a fairly high response rate at a very low cost. Nonrespondents were probably primarily students not in school on the day the questionnaires were administered. Although absenteeism is undoubtedly not a random phenomenon, the bias resulting from such nonresponse may be modest. To be on the safe side, Alongi would do well to try to administer the questionnaire to a subsample of absent students to determine the direction on any biases (if any). A more serious problem, however, is that Alongi's population appears to be defined as "urban adolescents." Because she distributed the questionnaires through the school system, adolescents who had dropped out of high school could not possibly have been included in the sample. This is an especially serious problem because high-school dropouts are probably at substantially greater risk of using drugs than are high-school students. Alongi should stipulate that her target population is urban high-school students.

Another reason for using an interview rather than a questionnaire is that one can typically get more detailed information in an interview through open-ended questions. In this study, the researcher focused primarily on descriptive information, which can easily be obtained by means of closed-ended questions. Alongi's use of primarily closed-ended questions seems appropriate in terms of her method of data collection because many students would not want to take the time to write out long essays in response to open-ended questions. However, it must be acknowledged that many interesting pieces of information about adolescent drug use would not be obtainable through a self-administered questionnaire. For example, the study would probably not shed much light on how the students started taking drugs, how they felt about their drug use, what (if anything) they had done to curtail their use, and so on.

Another risk that Alongi ran by using a questionnaire was that some students might have had reading problems; reading levels clearly are not a problem in an interview. Assuming that the researcher took care in using simple, clear questions and a well-formatted questionnaire, the use of a questionnaire in this study is probably still defensible, particularly given the other advantages of this method of data collection. One of the ways in which Alongi could have checked on the appropriateness of the questionnaire's reading level was through adequate pretesting. Her use of 10 college freshmen in the pretest was not justifiable. The ability of these 10 students to comprehend the questions would tell the researcher nothing about the ability of a ninth-grade student who had repeated two grades to understand the questions and how to answer them. Alongi should have administered the pretest to at least 20 to 25 high school students, making sure that the pretest sample included students with low reading skills.

In summary, Alongi's distribution of questionnaires to high school students was defensible, assuming the target population is more narrowly defined, and assuming the focus is primarily on drug use incidence. In this study, interviews would have been more problematic because the sample would likely have been smaller and candor might have been lower because responses would not be anonymous. The use of self-reports was also justifiable—no other method, in fact, seems very appropriate. Alongi's biggest data collection error was inadequate pretesting of the questionnaire.

D.4. Lovely constructed a Likert scale to measure nurses' attitudes toward abortion. Likert scales are the most widely used means of measuring attitudes, so Lovely's choice was understandable. With a 17-item scale, Lovely was able to make fine discriminations among people with different attitudes (scores could range from 17 to 119).

Each item on the scale consists of a declarative statement with which respondents are asked to agree or disagree. The scale consists of both positively and negatively worded statements in a seemingly random order of presentation. A careful reading of the statements, however, suggests that the researcher might have positive attitudes toward abortion rights: 11 of the 17 items in the final scale are worded positively, which could bias some people's responses. The researcher should either replace a couple of pro-choice statements with anti-abortion statements or should add two or three more anti-abortion statements.

One commendable aspect of Lovely's scale is that it is relatively long. A shortcoming of many Likert scales is that they are too short. A short scale often leads to unstable, unreliable results.

Lovely pretested her scale with 10 nurses. Generally, a larger sample would be advisable, especially if one were to take the recommended steps for estimating the scale's reliability and validity (not discussed in the textbook until Chapter 10). However, Lovely did well to do a pretest; some researchers fail to take even this precaution. The pretest apparently yielded some useful information because three items were eliminated. Judging from the items, their removal seems justified. They do not appear to be measures of attitudes toward abortion per se but rather toward other things. For example, item 3 is mostly a measure of political or fiscal attitudes. Lovely may have detected this problem by learning that several of the nurses with strong pro-choice attitudes nevertheless disagreed with this item. Question 6 might have been eliminated if all respondents, regardless of their attitudes toward abortion, tended to agree with it.

In summary, Lovely did a reasonable job in creating this Likert scale. Adding more anti-abortion items and pretesting the scale a second time would probably improve the scale. Conversely, one must wonder why Lovely created this scale from scratch, given the existence of many other scales that measure abortion attitudes.

D.5. Bingham collected data on parents' experiences in caring for their dying children through in-depth interviews and observations. By using an observational approach, the researcher was able to directly see the parents' caregiving behaviors rather than relying on their reports about their own behavior.

By using an unstructured approach, Bingham could explore the full range of the caretaking experience—not only what was being done but also what was being said, what was *not* being done, and what was being expressed nonverbally (*e.g.,* through body language, and so forth). In other words, an unstructured approach gave the researcher the opportunity to look at the experience holistically.

Although the observation was unstructured, the approach cannot be described as participant observation. That is, the researcher did not actually care for the sick children or engage in any other parenting behavior.

Clearly, the parents knew of the researcher's presence and knew of the purpose of the observations. It is therefore possible that reactivity was a problem—that is, that the parents' caregiving behaviors were altered because of the known presence of the researcher. However, it is commendable that the researcher made 10 observations of each family over a 2-month period. Undoubtedly, the reactivity problem would diminish over time as family members became more accustomed to having the researcher there. It is unlikely, though, that reactivity would disappear completely.

D.7. Van Vlieberghe chose a biophysiologic measure—hematocrit readings—to evaluate the effectiveness of her nutritional intervention with pregnant women. This choice was a good one for several reasons. First, as mentioned in the text, biophysiologic measures such as this one are objective, are not open to deliberate falsification because of the subject's desire to look good, and are relatively sensitive indicators of subject status. Because of the investigator's interest in analyzing *change* over the course of the intervention, the chosen measure was well suited in that it could not be influenced by a testing effect (*i.e.,* the administration of the hematocrit test at the 36-week measurement was completely independent of the influence of the previous measurement). The measures were unobtrusive in the sense that the subjects were not aware that the blood tests were being used to test Van Vlieberghe's research hypothesis that the intervention would decrease anemia (although not unobtrusive to the subjects in a general sense). Presumably, the use of hematocrit test results was also cost-effective.

Conversely, the use of the hematocrit readings alone yielded very little information about how (if at all) the intervention could be improved. The results suggested that the intervention did not have the desired effects; but this finding could reflect, for example, too small a sample or inadequate length of time between changes in nutritional habits and the final measurements. Additional data should probably have been collected to provide greater insights into the findings. In particular, Van Vlieberghe would have been wise to collect supplementary self-report data regarding the women's nutritional practices and attitudes. Observational data would also be desirable (*e.g.,* to see what types of food the subjects ate) and could perhaps have been obtained in a structured or staged setting but would be difficult to obtain on a day-to-day basis. Such measures would not necessarily be *preferred* to physiologic measures because of the issues raised in the paragraph above, but they would have greatly enhanced Van Vlieberghe's study if used as a supplement.

◩ TEST QUESTIONS AND ANSWERS

Multiple Choice

1. Which of the following types of research does *not* use existing data?
    a. Historical research
    b. Secondary analysis
    *c. Survey research
    d. Record-based research

2. Among which of the following dimensions do self-report methods vary?
    a. Structure
    b. Quantifiability
    c. Objectivity
    *d. All of the above

3. Which of the following data collection approaches does not belong with the others?
    *a. Questionnaire
    b. Focused interview
    c. Life history
    d. Focus group interview

4. A major advantage of fixed alternative questions is that they:
    a. Are easy to construct
    *b. Are analyzed in a straightforward manner
    c. Encourage in-depth responses
    d. All of the above

5. A major purpose of a pretest is to:
    *a. Detect inadequacies in an interview schedule or questionnaire
    b. Obtain some preliminary results on the research problem
    c. Assess the adequacy of the research design
    d. Evaluate whether a structured schedule is preferable

6. Interviews are generally preferable to questionnaires because:
    a. They are less expensive
    b. They are easier to analyze
    *c. The quality of the data tends to be higher
    d. There is less opportunity for bias

7. On a seven-point Likert scale, a person who neither agreed nor disagreed with the statement would be scored as:
    a. 0
    b. 1
    *c. 4
    d. 7

8. On a 20-item Likert scale with five response categories, the range of possible scores is:
    a. 0 to 100
    b. 20 to 80
    *c. 20 to 100
    d. 0 to 50

9. The semantic differential scale consists of:
   a. A series of declarative statements along an agree–disagree continuum
   b. A small number of test items on semantics
   c. Items that measure facts rather than attitudes
   *d. Sets of bipolar adjectives arranged along a continuum of degree of feeling about a concept

10. The social desirability response set is least likely to be a problem on scales incorporated into which of the following?
    *a. Mailed questionnaire
    b. Face-to-face interview
    c. Telephone interview
    d. All of the above are equivalent

11. The technique that is least susceptible to response-set bias is:
    a. Interviews
    b. Q sorts
    c. Questionnaires
    *d. Projective measures

12. Vignettes are often incorporated into:
    a. Focus group interviews
    *b. Questionnaires
    c. Observational rating scales
    d. Projective techniques

13. When an observer is not concealed, the findings may be biased because of:
    *a. Reactivity
    b. Ethical problems
    c. Lack of mobility
    d. Acquiescence response set

14. An observer who moves around the site to observe behaviors from different locations is using:
    a. Single positioning
    *b. Multiple positioning
    c. Mobile positioning
    d. None of the above

15. Which of the following structured observational methods records the degree of behavior observed along a continuum?
    a. Category system
    b. Sign system
    c. Checklist
    *d. Rating scale

16. In participant observation, data are collected in the form of:
    a. Checklists
    *b. Field notes
    c. Rating scales
    d. Sign systems

17. A sphygmomanometer yields:
    *a. An in vivo measure
    b. An in vitro measure
    c. Either an in vivo or in vitro measure
    d. None of the above

18. Which of the following is an example of an in vitro measure?
    a. Electromyogram recordings
    b. Thermistor readings
    *c. Stool cultures
    d. Renal arteriograms

True/False

(T)   1. When a researcher re-analyzes previously collected data, the study is often referred to as a secondary analysis.

(T)   2. Questionnaires tend to be high on structure, quantifiability, obtrusiveness, and objectivity.

(F)   3. Most nursing research studies involve data collected by structured biophysiologic measures.

(F)   4. The greater the degree of structure an interview has, the more accurate are the results.

(F)   5. Topic guides are used to collect data in unstructured observational studies.

(F)   6. Interview schedules tend to be more structured than questionnaires.

(T)   7. A major purpose of tightly structured questionnaires is to ensure comparability of responses from subjects.

(T)   8. Closed-ended questions ask participants to choose the most appropriate answer from a list of alternatives.

(F)   9. Open-ended items are more difficult to construct than closed-ended ones.

(F) 10. Interview schedules are generally more effective than questionnaires as a means of obtaining information about socially unacceptable behaviors.

(T) 11. Questionnaires should be pretested with people whose characteristics are similar to those of the eventual study participants.

(F) 12. One of the disadvantages of telephone interviews is the low response rate.

(F) 13. The most common type of scaling procedure used in attitude measurement is the semantic differential scale.

(T) 14. The values of negatively worded items should be reversed in scoring a Likert scale.

(F) 15. Sets of bipolar adjective pairs are characteristic of visual analog scales.

(T) 16. Response-set bias refers to a person's tendency to respond characteristically in a particular way, regardless of the item's content.

(F) 17. An advantage of using the Q-sort technique is its relative ease of administration.

(T) 18. One of the problems associated with projective techniques is uncertainties in the degree to which they measure the concept they purport to measure.

(F) 19. Participant observation is considered a structured type of observational method.

(T) 20. The researcher engages in activities of the group being studied in participant observation research.

(F) 21. Exhaustive category systems are sometimes referred to as sign systems.

(T) 22. Reactivity refers to changes in participants' behaviors due to the presence of an observer.

(T) 23. Biophysiologic measures may be used as either independent variables or dependent variables in a study.

(F) 24. One of the greatest strengths of biophysiologic measures is their unobtrusiveness.

Chapter 10
Data Quality Assessments

◪ STATEMENT OF INTENT

Chapter 10 is designed to assist students in evaluating data quality in research reports. Because quantitative data are collected in most nursing studies, the beginning section of the chapter introduces students to the basic principles of measurement; the characteristics of measurement are described, and the importance of measurement in the scientific process is explained. A major intent here is to have students recognize that quantitative measurement is neither inherent nor arbitrary and that good measuring tools have certain attributes for which the researcher is often responsible.

The subsequent section explains how measurement error can interfere with the accuracy of quantitative measurements and indicates several sources of measurement error. The concepts of reliability and validity are then dealt with in some detail. Both reliability and validity have multiple aspects, each of which can be assessed differently. It is important for the student to recognize, however, that for any given instrument, some ways of assessing reliability and validity are more appropriate than others. Another important point is that the quality of an instrument partially depends on its particular application.

Various criteria for evaluating qualitative data quality are also described, and techniques for enhancing and documenting the trustworthiness of qualitative data are reviewed. Students should be expected to realize, after reading this chapter, that qualitative and quantitative researchers are equally interested in having their data reflect reality as accurately and truthfully as possible. Even though the terminology for assessments of quantitative and qualitative data is different, the underlying concepts are similar. All researchers have the responsibility of persuading consumers of research reports that their findings are worthy of confidence, and consumers need to carefully attend to the evidence that data quality merits such confidence when reading research reports.

COMMENTS ON THE ACTUAL RESEARCH EXAMPLES IN THE TEXTBOOK

Quantitative Research Example: A Structured Scale

Prescott and colleagues (1991) undertook a psychometric assessment of the Patient Intensity for Nursing Index (PINI), a tool for the identification of nursing resource consumption in acute care settings. Below are several comments on the researchers' activities.

- The researchers undertook two methods of testing the reliability of the PINI, both of which were appropriate approaches, given the nature of the scale. First, they evaluated the degree of internal consistency among the 10 items on the PINI and found that the homogeneity of the items was fairly high ($r = .85$).

- Next, the researchers evaluated the extent to which two independent nurses using the PINI would assign similar scores for the same patient. Because the PINI involves many items that are judgmental and subjective, interrater reliability was the most important type of reliability to assess. Their method of assessing interrater reliability was efficient; it involved having two different nurses (the day shift and evening shift nurses) rate the patient as close in time as possible. Unfortunately, approximately 4 hours typically elapsed between the ratings. Therefore, the interrater reliability could have been depressed by *real* differences in the patients' status over time. Of course, this difficulty could only have been overcome if each patient simultaneously had two nurses, each of whom did a rating, but this could have confounded the ratings in other ways and would have been costly and impractical. The overall interrater reliability of .61 is respectable but perhaps suggests the need for additional training in use of the PINI.

- The researchers did not describe the actual development of the PINI in their 1991 research report, so the extent to which they strove to make the scale content valid is unknown.

- The researchers undertook a series of excellent substudies to test the validity of the PINI. First, it is noteworthy that the validity testing took place in five geographically dispersed hospitals. Moreover, 29 clinical units, including various types of units, were used to draw a large sample of nurses (487) and patients (more than 6000). (Although not mentioned in the textbook, the researchers also took care to exclude from the sample outliers—patients who were hospitalized for more than 1 month.)

- The substudies involved activities that could be described as offering evidence of both criterion-related and construct-related validity. With respect to criterion-related validity, Prescott and her colleagues tested the relationship between PINI scores and six other concurrent criteria, such as the patients' length of hospital stay. In all cases, the correlations were significant, and in several cases, they were quite substantial (*e.g.*, the correlation between PINI scores and the MEDICUS classification system was .70). The researchers also correlated nurses' ratings on one item of the PINI (hours of care) with the ratings of independent observers on this same dimension. Although the researchers referred to this as a validity substudy, it represents another effort to determine interrater reliability—that is, the *accuracy* of the nurses' estimates of the hours of care provided to the patient. Here the researchers found that agreement was fairly high (69%) but improvable.

- With respect to construct validity, the factor analysis identified three independent dimensions of the PINI, which confirmed two of the researchers' four a priori dimensions: severity and complexity. The most important evidence of the PINI's construct validity comes from the researchers' use of the known-groups procedure. They contrasted low nursing intensity and high nursing intensity groups (as categorized on the basis of diagnostic-related groups) and found strikingly different PINI scores ($p < .0001$). Thus, overall, the researchers were able to marshal substantial evidence that the PINI is reliable and valid.

Qualitative Research Example

Gagliardi (1991) collected a considerable amount of qualitative data regarding the experience of families living with a child with Duchenne muscular dystrophy. Below are a few comments regarding Gagliardi's efforts to enhance, appraise, and describe data quality.

- Gagliardi documented, to a far greater degree than is typical in qualitative studies, the steps she took to improve and evaluate data quality. Her report could serve as a model of the kinds of information consumers should look for and expect in a qualitative study.

- Gagliardi used many of the techniques suggested by Lincoln and Guba. Triangulation of various types were used to converge on the truth. First, method triangulation was used: the study used both in-depth interviews and personal observations to understand how the lives of family members were affected by the presence of a Duchenne child. Second, multiple sources of data were obtained (data triangulation): the researcher interviewed multiple family members in each family and made observations in a variety of contexts. Finally, the assistance of colleagues allowed the researcher to use investigator triangulation in the categorization of collected data. Moreover, reported rates of agreement were high, and debriefings helped the researcher to identify possible biases in her understanding of the data.

- Gagliardi also used member checks to verify the accuracy of her interpretation of the data. In two rounds of follow-up interviews, she asked family members to validate the merit of the emerging themes that she had identified.

- Gagliardi went considerably further in establishing the worth of her data than most qualitative researchers by having two external reviewers audit her work. Her audit trail included her logs, her analytic memoranda (which themselves recorded possible biases noted by the researcher herself), and transcribed interviews.
- Although Gagliardi's efforts are exemplary, there is at least one way in which the quality of her data might have been improved. She spent only 1 day per week for 10 weeks in the field. This level of engagement seems relatively brief and might not have been sufficient for the family members to let down their defenses—that is, to act naturally in the presence of the observer or to candidly discuss their feelings and concerns in the interviews.

◼ ANSWERS TO SELECTED STUDY-GUIDE EXERCISES

A.1.
1. a
2. c
3. b
4. c
5. a
6. d
7. b
8. a

A.2.
1. a
2. c
3. b
4. d
5. a
6. b

B.
1. Attributes (characteristics)
2. Quantification
3. Rules
4. True score
5. Measurement error
6. True score
7. Stability
8. Split-half
9. Homogeneity
10. Interrater (interobserver) reliability
11. Valid
12. Face
13. Content
14. Predictive
15. Credibility, transferability, dependability, confirmability
16. Prolonged engagement
17. Data triangulation
18. Member checking
19. Confirmability
20. Inquiry audit

D.2. Gardner constructed a 10-item scale to measure paternal bonding in new fathers. To assess the scale's reliability, she used the split-half technique, which assesses the internal consistency of an instrument. Gardner's focus on the homogeneity of the items in the scale was appropriate. It would probably make little sense to assess the scale's stability over time; paternal bonding may well change on a daily basis, so modest correlations between two administrations of the scale would not necessarily reflect unreliability but rather true change in the attribute being measured. The equivalence aspect of reliability also is not relevant here. Thus, Gardner did well to focus on internal consistency, but she would have obtained more accurate reliability estimates using Cronbach's alpha method.

Gardner's computations indicate that the reliability of the scale could and should be improved. With a reliability coefficient of .62, there is considerable measurement error. The easiest way to improve the reliability of this scale would be to add more items. Other techniques, such as those noted in the discussion of the fictitious example in the textbook, could also be used to determine if items on the scale should be discarded or revised.

Two methods were used to evaluate the scale's validity. The content validity approach was useful and provided important information, though in itself, content validation could not be said to demonstrate that the new scale was valid. Gardner's second approach to validation, unfortunately, had other problems. She used criterion-related validity, with nurses' ratings used as the criterion against which the fathers' scale scores were compared. One major problem here is that the validity of the nurses' ratings themselves is questionable. The most defensible aspect of validity on which to focus in this case is construct validity. The known-groups technique might have been used by a comparison of scores of, for example, new fathers and fathers of 6-month-old infants (one would expect paternal bonding to be higher in the latter group).

The validity coefficient obtained by correlating father's scores with nurses' ratings tells us very little. First, there is an upper ceiling on the validity coefficient because of the low reliability of the scale. Second, a poor validity coefficient could also reflect the low reliability and validity of the nurses' ratings. Gardner should scrutinize each item on the original scale for its ability to contribute to the scale's reliability, add items to the revised scale, readminister the longer scale to a new sample, and then use a construct validation approach in estimating the scale's validity.

▨ TEST QUESTIONS AND ANSWERS

Multiple Choice

1. The difference between a true score and an obtained score is referred to as:

    a. Internal inconsistency   c. Response sampling
    b. Triangulation   *d. Error of measurement

2. One source of measurement error is:

    *a. Response-set bias   c. Inquiry audits
    b. Obtained scores   d. Homogeneity

3. Cronbach's alpha is used to determine which of the following instrument attributes?

    *a. Internal consistency   c. Criterion validity

    b. Stability   d. Construct validity

4. The aspect of reliability for which interobserver reliability is appropriate is:

    a. Stability   *c. Equivalence

    b. Internal consistency   d. Criterion-related

5. The type of validity that employs logical rather than empirical procedures in its assessment is:

    *a. Content   c. Predictive

    b. Concurrent   d. Construct

6. Suppose a researcher were interested in assessing the adequacy of an instrument to measure the concept of hopelessness. The type of validation procedure would most probably be:

    a. Content   c. Predictive

    b. Concurrent   *d. Construct

7. Which of the following terms does not belong with the other three?

    *a. Content validity   c. Predictive validity

    b. Criterion-related validity   d. Concurrent validity

8. If unstructured interviews and observations both were used to collect data on a single construct in one study, this would be referred to as:

    a. Data triangulation   c. Theory triangulation

    b. Investigator triangulation   *d. Method triangulation

9. A member check involves reviewing data with:

    a. An external auditor   *c. An informant or person being observed

    b. A peer of the researcher   d. A second member of the research team

10. The criterion that refers to the neutrality of qualitative data is:

    a. Credibility   c. Dependability

    b. Transferability   *d. Confirmability

11. The use of prolonged engagement in the collection of qualitative data enhances which of the following?

    *a. Credibility of the data   c. Dependability of the data

    b. Transferability of the data   d. Confirmability of the data

12. An overall assessment of the adequacy of a structured self-report or observational instrument is referred to as a:

    a. Triangulation study   c. Construct validation

    *b. Psychometric evaluation   d. Measurement critique

True/False

(T) 1. Measurement may be defined as the assignment of numbers to characteristics of objects according to specified rules.

(T) 2. A good measurement tool results in a quantitative score for a single attribute of the object being measured.

(T) 3. A major purpose of measurement is to differentiate between objects that possess varying amounts of the trait being studied.

(F) 4. Reliability refers to the extent to which an instrument measures the concept that the researcher thinks is being measured.

(T) 5. A reliable measure is one that minimizes the error component of an obtained score.

(F) 6. Comparing the odd-numbered and even-numbered responses of a person on a test is an example of test–retest reliability.

(F) 7. An instrument can be valid even when it is not reliable.

(F) 8. If an instrument had a criterion-related validity coefficient of .54, a researcher should conclude that the tool was both unreliable and not valid.

(T) 9. No numeric index is obtained for content validity.

(T) 10. An achievement test that is high on content validity can nevertheless yield scores with considerable measurement error.

(F) 11. Conceptually, methods of assessing the quality of quantitative and qualitative data are totally distinct.

(T) 12. Data triangulation involves collecting similar information on the topics of interest from multiple sources.

(F) 13. An inquiry audit is usually performed by members of the research team.

(T) 14. Dependability of qualitative data is to the stability/reliability of a quantitative measure what confirmability (qualitative) is to equivalence/reliability (quantitative).

(F) 15. Evidence of the trustworthiness of qualitative data is routinely provided in research reports.

Analysis of Research Data

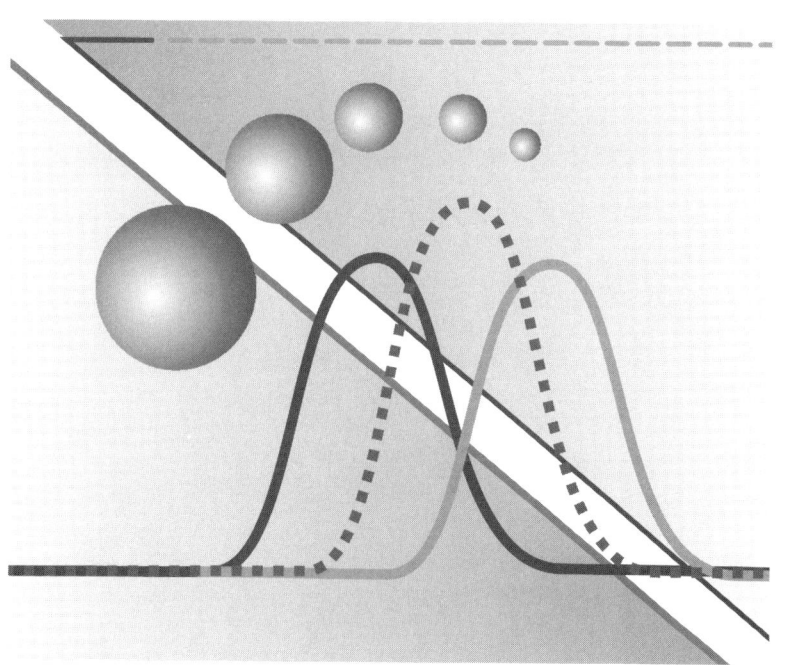

PART V

Chapter 11
Quantitative Analysis

◩ STATEMENT OF INTENT

Chapter 11 introduces students to some basic principles of quantitative analysis. The chapter covers materials that are typically covered in a full-year course of statistics, but the emphasis throughout is not on computation or on understanding fundamental principles of probability. Rather, the focus is on helping consumers of nursing research studies understand how and why certain statistical procedures are used and on helping them understand and interpret statistics reported in research reports.

The chapter begins with a description of the four levels of measurement, followed by a discussion of elementary descriptive statistics. The chapter covers the three basic types of univariate descriptive statistics (description of the shape of a distribution, central tendency, and variability) and methods of bivariate statistics.

The next major section discusses the fundamental principles underlying tests of statistical significance. A major aim is to show students *why* inferential statistics are needed to draw conclusions about research data. As in the previous section, the discussion focuses not on calculations but rather on the logic, use, and interpretation of various statistics. In fact, in this edition *all* computations, formulas, and Greek symbols have been omitted. The tests described in the chapter include *t*-tests, analysis of variance, chi-squared tests, and product–moment correlation coefficients.

The chapter also presents some preliminary information about multivariate statistical procedures. Increasing numbers of nurse researchers are using sophisticated multivariate statistical procedures to analyze their data, and even beginning students are likely to be faced with studies in which such a procedure was used. Chapter 11 tries to familiarize readers with some of these procedures and illustrates how and when they are used. The procedures include multiple regression, analysis of covariance, and factor analysis, with brief mention of a discriminant function analysis, multivariate ANOVA, and logistic regression.

The chapter concludes with some tips on how to read and evaluate the results section of a quantitative research report.

◪ COMMENTS ON THE ACTUAL RESEARCH EXAMPLES IN THE TEXTBOOK

Example of Descriptive Statistics

Gray and colleagues (1995) used a variety of descriptive statistics to describe their data. Here are a few comments on their analysis.

- The researchers used descriptive statistics to describe the characteristics of their sample—specifically their age, gender, and cause of the spinal cord injury. Gray and colleagues used measures of central tendency (*e.g.,* mean age), as well as of variability (age ranges). However, the researchers could in some instances have been more specific. For example, although they indicated that the most common (modal) cause of the spinal cord injury was motor vehicle accident, they did not indicate the actual percentage, and thus readers do not know whether accidents caused 40% or 90% of the injuries. It is also somewhat surprising that no information was presented about other characteristics of the sample (*e.g.,* their race/ethnicity, socioeconomic status, etc.).
- All of the findings of the report regarding the incidence and characteristics of urinary incontinence were presented as frequencies, percentages, or modes. Given the nature of the data and the descriptive intent of the study, this was appropriate. Most of the key study variables were nominal-level variables. For example, having versus not having any incontinent episodes is a nominal-level variable. Other variables were ordinal-level, with only a few categories (*e.g.,* volume of leakage was measured as minimal, moderate, or large).
- It is not clear from the report whether the data were *gathered* as nominal/ordinal variables, or converted after the fact. For example, the researchers reported that 85% of the sample experienced one or more symptomatic urinary tract infection. If the researchers asked study participants to report the *actual* number of infections experienced, they could also have reported the mean number of infections for the sample. If, however, subjects were given response alternatives such as "none; one; two or more," then a mean could not have been computed.
- Graphs were used effectively to highlight a few of the more noteworthy findings. It is possible that a table could have been used to more concisely summarize some of the major findings.

Example of Bivariate Inferential Statistics

Lattavo and her colleagues (1995) conducted an interesting study designed to compare core pulmonary artery temperature measures with other types of temperature measures. Here are a few comments about their study.

- The researchers first used Pearson product–moment correlation coefficients to examine the direction and intensity of relationship between core PA and all other temperature measurements. The temperatures were all interval-level measures, and so it was appropriate to compute correlation coefficients.
- The findings showed that all correlations were moderately high, and significantly different from zero—that is, that there is a true relationship between the temperature measures and not just a relationship that happened by chance in this particular sample. However, the correlation coefficients were not as substantial as might be considered ideal if one measure were being used as a substitute for the other. For example, the correlation between axillary temperature and core PA temperature was only .68, meaning that less than half of the variance in these two measures is shared ($r^2 = .46$).
- The researcher established a criterion of .80 as the amount of shared variance needed to conclude that alternative measures were reliable substitutes for core PA temperature measures. This is a fairly arbitrary criterion, but it is nevertheless a reasonable one. Moreover, the researchers substantiated their conclusions by performing paired t-tests.
- The use of paired rather than independent groups t-tests was appropriate, because the measures were from the same subjects. In these t-tests, the dependent variable was the interval-level temperature measure and the independent variable was type of measurement (*e.g.,* core PA versus tympanic). Strictly speaking, however, the use of a series of paired t-tests was not appropriate: a repeated measures ANOVA would have been preferable because there were five separate temperature measurements. Multiple t-tests increases the risk of a Type I error. However, the t-tests were fairly consistent in indicating that core PA temperature measures were significantly different from other types of temperature measures. It seems highly likely that the researchers came to the correct conclusion based on their analysis.
- Although studies that use bivariate statistics can often be strengthened through the use of multivariate procedures, it is not clear in this study what could have been gained by using multivariate statistics. For example, ANCOVA might have been used to control extraneous variables, but with subjects serving as their own controls, all background characteristics were automatically controlled through the research design.

Example of Multivariate Statistical Analysis

Kocher and Thomas (1994) conducted a study with a strong sampling design and then used several sophisticated analytic procedures. The following comments focus mainly on their statistical analyses.

- ■ The researchers were interested in identifying factors that could predict the retention of nurses in the Army. Their predictor variables included demographic background variables (*e.g.,* marital status, race), characteristics of the external job market, and 10 job satisfaction questions. Laudably, the researchers began with an effort to make the prediction equation more streamlined, that is, reduce the number of predictors.
- ■ The researchers used factor analysis to determine the underlying dimensionality of the 10 job satisfaction items. Although factor analysis is usually performed with more than 10 variables, this analysis appears to have been successful in reducing job satisfaction to four independent dimensions.
- ■ The primary analysis was logistic regression, which is the appropriate analysis when the dependent variable is nominal-level. In this case, the dependent variable was job retention (nurse remained versus did not remain on active duty). The independent variables were a combination of nominal-level variables (*e.g.,* marital status), interval-level variables (*e.g.,* scores on the "work/military life" job satisfaction scale); and ratio-level variables (*e.g.,* age). Note that in this situation, discriminant analysis could also have been used; the conclusions would likely have been identical.
- ■ Because a multivariate procedure was used, the researchers were able to conclude that two dimensions of job satisfaction were significant predictors of retention *even when* demographic characteristics were controlled. If a bivariate procedure (*e.g.,* *t*-tests) had been used to compare retained and nonretained nurses on job satisfaction dimensions, the researchers would not have known if the dimensions were confounded with background characteristics.

▨ ANSWERS TO SELECTED STUDY-GUIDE EXERCISES

A.1.

1.	d	7.	b
2.	a	8.	d
3.	d	9.	c
4.	b	10.	b
5.	c	11.	c
6.	a	12.	a

A.2.

1.	b	6.	b
2.	a	7.	b
3.	c	8.	a
4.	c	9.	c
5.	d	10.	a

A.3.

1. b	6. a
2. a	7. a
3. d	8. a
4. b	9. d
5. c	10. c

A.4.

1. a, b, d	5. a, b, c, d, e
2. a	6. b, d
3. c	7. d
4. e	8. e

B.

1. Enumeration (count)
2. Ordinal
3. Zero
4. Equal distances
5. Parameter
6. Frequency distribution
7. Frequency polygons
8. Symmetric
9. Negatively
10. Unimodal
11. Normal curve (bell-shaped curve)
12. Central tendency
13. Variability
14. Homogeneous
15. Standard deviation
16. Bivariate statistics
17. Negative (inverse)
18. Pearson's r (product–moment correlation coefficient)
19. Inferential statistics
20. Normal
21. Type I
22. Parametric
23. Levels of significance
24. Type II
25. F-ratio
26. Chi-squared test
27. R
28. Analysis of covariance
29. Covariate
30. Factors
31. Factor extraction phase
32. Multivariate analysis of variance

C.3. Unimodal, fairly symmetric

C.4. Mean: 81.13; Median: 83; Mode: 84

C.7.

a. Chi-squared
b. t-test
c. Pearson's r
d. ANOVA

C.9.

a. Discriminant function analysis or logistic regression
b. ANCOVA
c. MANOVA
d. Multiple regression

D.2. The following is a list of all the variables in Bentley's study and the level of measurement for each:

absence or presence of sleep prob-lems	nominal
amount of anesthesia	ordinal
time spent in labor	ratio
type of delivery	nominal
birth weight	ratio
Apgar score	interval

The six variables in the research covered all four levels of measurement. Most of the variables were measured on the highest possible scale, but in two instances, a higher level was possible. The first was the dependent variable, sleep-disturbance problems. An infant could be rated in terms of the degree of sleeping problems; such ratings would yield at least ordinal and perhaps interval data. Alternatively, one could use a more objective measure of sleeping behavior, such as the number of consecutive hours of sleep per night, the number of nocturnal sleep interruptions, or the number of changes from sleep to wake states per day. All these would yield ratio-level data.

The second variable that could be measured on a higher level is the amount of anesthesia used at delivery. Here, the actual amount could be measured. It would probably be worthwhile to separate different types of anesthesia administered as well. Changes such as those suggested could, in fact, alter Bentley's findings and conclusions.

D.4. Langevin appropriately used a variety of quantitative descriptive statistics for the data he collected. (Some might argue that he should have collected in-depth qualitative data instead of, or in addition to, the quantitative information, given the nature of his research question.)

Langevin used all five major types of descriptive statistics discussed in Chapter 10, as follows:

Frequency distribution	Self-ratings of health
Central tendency	Predicted length of stay (mean and median)
Variability	Predicted length of stay (standard deviation)
Contingency table	Mobility group by self-ratings of health
Correlation	Predicted length of stay and self-ratings of health

Langevin's selection of statistics generally seems appropriate for the level of measurement of the variables. For example, predicted length of stay was measured on a ratio scale; means and standard deviations are suitable. Langevin also reported a median for this variable, and, although not necessary, this information would suggest to an alert reader that the distribution is skewed. The self-rating, in contrast, is an ordinal-level variable. Summarizing the data on this variable by means of a frequency distribution was acceptable, although the medians also could have been computed. Similarly, rather than constructing a contingency table for this variable, Langevin could have computed medians for each of the three groups. However, Langevin's method is not really wrong—many researchers summarize ordinal data by use of percentages.

Langevin's presentation communicated considerable information in a short amount of space. Langevin's data consisted of 240 values organized and integrated into a concise summary. His statement suggests that his hypothesis has some support, although inferential statistics would be needed to verify this. High-mobility patients were three times as likely to rate themselves as being healthy as were low-mobility patients. Increased mobility was also associated with fewer predicted days of hospitalization. Interestingly, variability also increased as the means increased. The high-mobility group generally agreed that their length of hospital stay would be short. In the low-mobility group, however, some patients predicted fairly short stays, whereas others thought they would be there over a month. We would have had more information on this point if Langevin has also presented the ranges for this variable for the three groups.

D.6. Kuhara had five dependent variables, all of which were measured on an interval scale. Her independent variable, age, was measured on a nominal scale, although it could have been measured on a ratio scale using actual ages rather than age ranges. Had Kuhara used actual ages, five Pearson's r statistics could have been computed to summarize the magnitude of the relationship between age and the five test scores.

One of the difficulties of using correlational procedures, however, is that these statistics can only describe and test linear relationships (wherein the values are in a straight ascending or descending order). In the current example, the relationship between age and test scores is reasonably, but not completely, linear. For the salty test, for example, test scores decline as age increases; for the sweet test, however, the 51- to 60-year-old group has the highest scores. ANOVA procedures, which were used in this case, have the advantage of communicating a lot of information about trends in the data. The researcher could have computed a correlational statistic (preferably Pearson's r with actual age data) in addition to the ANOVA.

The table shows that there were 3 and 76 degrees of freedom (df), which is correct (4 groups minus 1 = 3; 80 subjects minus 4 groups = 76).

The results suggest that age is only weakly related to taste acuity. Only in the case of salty substances was there a significant decline with age. All other observed differences could have been the result of chance. However, the differences *might* be real; a Type II error (rejecting a false null hypothesis) might have been committed. The *F* values for the bitter and overall test were fairly close to achieving statistical significance. Kuhara would do well to replicate her study using a larger sample and increasing the number of substances tested.

▧ TEST QUESTIONS AND ANSWERS

Multiple Choice

1. The level of measurement that classifies and ranks objects in terms of the degree to which they possess the attribute of interest is:
   - a. Nominal
   - *b. Ordinal
   - c. Interval
   - d. Ratio

2. Religion is measured on the:
   - *a. Nominal scale
   - b. Ordinal scale
   - c. Interval scale
   - d. Ratio scale

3. Which of the two variables—temperature in Fahrenheit degrees or weight in kilograms—uses a higher level of measurement?
   - a. Temperature in Fahrenheit degrees
   - *b. Weight in kilograms
   - c. Both are the same
   - d. Insufficient information to make a determination

4. A record of the fluid intake, in ounces, of a postsurgical patient is an example of which level of measurement?
   - a. Nominal
   - b. Ordinal
   - c. Interval
   - *d. Ratio

5. Which level of measurement permits the researcher to add, subtract, multiply, and divide?
   - a. Nominal
   - b. Ordinal
   - c. Interval
   - *d. Ratio

6. It is not meaningful to calculate an average with data from which of the following?
   - a. Nominal measures
   - b. Ordinal measures
   - *c. Nominal and ordinal measures
   - d. None of the above

7. Degrees such as associate's, bachelor's, master's, and doctorate correspond to measures on which of the following scales?
   - a. Nominal
   - *b. Ordinal
   - c. Interval
   - d. Ratio

8. If the bulk of scores from a test occurred at the upper end of the distribution, the distribution could be described as:
   - a. Normal
   - b. Bimodal
   - c. Positively skewed
   - *d. Negatively skewed

9. A group of 100 students took a test. The mean was 85, the standard deviation was 5, and the scores were normally distributed. About how many scores fell between 80 and 90?

  a. 40   c. 95

  *b. 68   d. Impossible to determine

10. A parameter is a characteristic of:

  *a. A population   c. A sample

  b. A frequency distribution   d. A normal curve

11. The mode is an index of:

  a. Bivariate relationships   c. Skewness

  *b. Central tendency   d. Variability

12. The measure of variability that takes into account all score values is the:

  a. Range   c. Mean

  b. Median   *d. Standard deviation

13. The measure of central tendency that is most stable is the:

  a. Mode   *c. Mean

  b. Median   d. They are all equivalent

14. If a variable were measured on a nominal scale, the most appropriate measure of central tendency would be the:

  *a. Mode   c. Mean

  b. Median   d. They are all equivalent

15. Which of the following is an example of a bivariate descriptive statistic?

  a. Frequency distribution   c. Range

  b. Mean   *d. Correlation coefficient

16. One of the characteristics of a normal distribution is that:

  a. It is bimodal   c. The values are positively

  *b. 68% of the values are within   skewed

    one standard deviation above   d. The mean is 50

    and below the mean

17. The symbol $\bar{\bar{X}}$ represents:

  a. The standard deviation   c. The total sample size

  *b. The mean   d. An individual score

18. The use of inferential statistics permits the researcher to:

  *a. Generalize to a population   c. Interpret descriptive statistics

    based on information gath-   d. None of the above

    ered from a sample

  b. Describe information obtained

    from empirical observation

19. The standard deviation of a sampling distribution is called a:

  a. Sampling error   c. Variance

  *b. Standard error   d. Parameter

20. The steps involved in using test statistics include all of the following *except*:

a. Determining the appropriate statistic to be used

b. Selecting a level of significance

c. Determining the degrees of freedom

*d. Calculating the theoretical distribution

21. A major factor that affects the standard error of the mean is the:

a. Value of the score range

b. Sampling distribution

*c. Sample size

d. Value of the mean

22. For which of the following levels of significance is the risk of making a Type II error greatest?

a. .10

b. .05

c. .01

*d. .001

23. If a researcher calculated a *t*-statistic to be −2.2 and the tabled *t* value (for a *df* of 60 and level of significance of .05) is 2.0, the researcher would:

a. Conclude that an error in calculation had been made

b. Accept the null hypothesis

*c. Reject the null hypothesis

d. Use a different level of significance

24. A statistical procedure that is used to determine whether a significant difference exists between any number of group means on a dependent variable measured on an interval scale is the:

a. *t*-test

*b. ANOVA

c. MANOVA

d. Factor analysis

25. How many null hypotheses would there be for a study with 40 subjects, using a two-way ANOVA?

a. 2

*b. 3

c. 5

d. 10

26. If a researcher wanted to determine whether observed proportions differed significantly from expected proportions, the statistic would be a(n):

a. *t*-test

b. Correlation coefficient

c. Analysis of variance

*d. Chi-squared test

27. When both the independent and dependent variables are measured on a ratio scale, the appropriate test statistic is a(n):

a. *t*-test

b. ANOVA

c. Chi-squared test

*d. Pearson's *r*

28. Suppose a researcher found a correlation of .40 between candy intake and dental caries. The amount of variability that could be accounted for in dental caries by candy intake is:

*a. 16%

b. 40%

c. 60%

d. None of the above

29. The multivariate procedure that reduces a large set of data into a more compact set of measures is:

    a. MANOVA

    *b. Factor analysis

    c. ANOVA

    d. Multiple regression

30. In analysis of covariance, a covariate is generally:

    a. An independent variable

    b. The dependent variable

    c. Either an independent or dependent variable

    *d. An extraneous variable

True/False

(F) 1. Researchers use descriptive statistics to draw conclusions about population values.

(F) 2. The type of graph that depicts the relation between two or more variables is called a frequency polygon.

(F) 3. A descriptive index from a population is called a statistic.

(T) 4. A frequency distribution is a systematic arrangement of scores according to the number of times each occurred.

(T) 5. The three characteristics that can completely summarize a set of data are the shape of the distribution, central tendency, and variability.

(F) 6. "Age at death" is an example of a positively skewed attribute.

(F) 7. The median is affected by the value of each individual score.

(T) 8. The standard deviation is a measure that tells how spread out scores are in a distribution.

(F) 9. Two sets of data with identical means would likely have the same standard deviation.

(T) 10. The standard deviation represents the average of the deviations from the mean.

(F) 11. A +.50 correlation coefficient indicates a stronger relationship than does a correlation of −.75.

(F) 12. Contingency tables are normally constructed with variables measured on the interval scale.

(F) 13. The tendency for statistical values to differ from one sample to another is known as the standard error of the mean.

(F) 14. As sample size decreases, so does the standard error of the mean.

(F) 15. A Type I error refers to the researcher's concluding that no difference exists when, in fact, a difference does exist.

(T) 16. A researcher never knows whether an error has been committed in statistical decision making.

(T) 17. A statistically significant finding means that the obtained results are not likely to have been due to chance.

(F) 18. Parametric tests make no assumptions about the shape of the distribution in the population.

(T) 19. The t-test is an example of a parametric statistical procedure.

(F) 20. It would be appropriate for a researcher to test the difference between the means of three groups of students by a t-test for independent samples.

(T) 21. Nonparametric tests have fewer assumptions than parametric tests.

(F) 22. The chi-squared statistic may be considered to be both descriptive and inferential.

(F) 23. The square root of a correlation coefficient tells how much variability in the dependent variable can be explained by the independent variable.

(T) 24. Variables are *not* classified as independent or dependent in factor analysis.

(F) 25. Discriminant analysis reduces a large set of data into a more manageable and meaningful form.

(T) 26. The dependent variable is measured on the nominal scale in discriminant function analysis.

(F) 27. In the following statement of results, the df stands for "direct F-ratio": $F = 5.2$, $df = 1,55$, $p < .05$.

(T) 28. In the following statement of results, the results are not statistically significant at conventional levels: ($r = .12$, $df = 33$, $p > .05$).

Chapter 12
The Analysis of Qualitative Data

▨ STATEMENT OF INTENT

The purpose of Chapter 12 is to acquaint students with some of the fundamental principles of analyzing narrative data from unstructured interviews and observations, as well as from written documents such as diaries and letters. The chapter begins by discussing the aims of qualitative research and describing the challenges that qualitative data analysts face. The next section discusses four major analysis styles that range on a continuum from standardized and systematic to intuitive and interpretive.

Although the results of qualitative analysis are usually easy for students to understand, it is often difficult to comprehend the *process* of the analysis—particularly because there are no firmly established rules. For this reason, the chapter devotes a disproportionate amount of time discussing the methods associated with grounded theory, about which a considerable amount has been written. Some basic procedures that are typically used for analyzing qualitative data are also presented, but these are not described in detail. The important point to emphasize is that the analysis of qualitative data is an inductively driven process that typically uses an iterative approach of gleaning meaning from the data and checking that meaning back against the data and against the interpretation of others, including the informants.

▨ COMMENTS ON THE ACTUAL RESEARCH EXAMPLES IN THE TEXTBOOK

Example of a Grounded Theory Study

Bright's (1992) study of the intergenerational context of a birth has many strong points as well as a few limitations. Here are a few comments regarding this study.

- The report described the process of data collection, coding, and data analysis in considerable detail. Consumers are given ample opportunity to evaluate the methods the researcher used.

- The data used in the analyses were obtained from multiple sources, including audiotaped interviews, videotaped interactions, and field notes from the researcher's observations of family activities and events.
- Because the analysis was ongoing, the researcher had the flexibility to follow up on hunches in subsequent interviews with family members and to obtain specific types of data needed to evaluate the adequacy of her hypotheses.
- The analysis style used in this study can best be described as an editing style. Constant comparison was used to continually refine and discard emerging hypotheses.
- Themes emerging from the data were subjected to verification by some of the sample members. A family therapist was asked to code a portion of the data. Both of these activities contributed to the trustworthiness of the data.
- Consistent with the grounded theory approach, Bright's analysis resulted in a theory that was grounded in her data. The theory concerned the basic social process of "making a place" for the infant.
- The use of only three families makes it difficult to know whether the social processes that Bright's analysis showed are idiosyncratic to these particular families. Even though Bright specifically sampled three families in which there was variation in terms of whether the pregnancy was intended, there are reasons to be cautious about the conclusions. This is particularly true because an increasing number of families do not have the kind of structure exemplified in these families—that is, with a husband and a wife and both sets of grandparents living nearby.
- The researcher made no mention of whether data saturation occurred. It appears as though the interviews might have been terminated at an arbitrary point (1 year after the child's birth) rather than at a theoretically meaningful point, although this may not be the case.
- Bright's report does not contain any excerpts from the interviews. Such excerpts are often useful in helping to give readers a stronger sense of the validity of the conclusions.

Example of an Analysis from an Ethnographic Study

Russell's (1996) ethnographic study resulted in a voluminous amount of data that needed to be analyzed. Here are a few comments regarding her qualitative analysis.

- Russell gathered a variety of data from different sources, which enabled her to get divergent perspectives on elders' care-seeking behavior. In addition to method triangulation, Russell used a strategy of prolonged engagement (*i.e.,* lengthy fieldwork) to enhance the credibility of her data.
- Russell collected and analyzed her data simultaneously, which gave her opportunities to gain insights into the types of data she needed to enhance her analysis.

- Like most qualitative researchers in this era, Russell used a computer to organize and manage her voluminous data.
- Russell's study is ethnographic, but it is difficult to draw conclusions about the overall analysis style. The codebook she developed could be interpreted as a template (*i.e.,* template analysis style) or as a categorization scheme as part of an editing analysis style. Many of the ways in which Russell described her analysis suggest some methods derived from grounded theory.
- Russell's analysis suggested a two-phase process with multiple stages in each. Her report used several excerpts from participant observation notes and interviews to illustrate and substantiate her interpretation of that process.

▧ ANSWERS TO SELECTED STUDY-GUIDE EXERCISES

A.

1. a	4. a
2. d	5. b
3. c	6. b

B.

1. Simultaneously
2. Comprehending, synthesizing, theorizing, recontextualizing
3. Indexing, categorizing
4. Constant comparison
5. Open coding (Level I coding)
6. Conceptual file
7. Computer programs
8. Themes
9. Quasi-statistics
10. Analytic induction
11. Axial coding
12. Basic social process

D.1. Crootof collected data on the experiences of patients who were on precautions. A qualitative approach was appropriate for the phenomenon being studied. Because the focus of the research was on patients' perspectives, direct observation and unstructured interviewing were reasonable methods of data collection. The researcher might have used more in-depth interviewing as data collection progressed; she also might have quantified her observations to determine the frequency of occurrence of relevant behaviors and incidents.

A time sampling plan was used in the observations. Observational periods spanned days, evenings, and nights. Crootof might have chosen to randomly sample the various times at which data would be collected rather than adhering to a rigid structure. A random procedure might have reduced any reactivity. A random observation plan would have made it more difficult for hospital staff to plan the times of their interactions. Although reactivity would probably still have been present, it might have been reduced.

Crootof recorded her observations after each 2-hour observation segment. It is not clear from the study summary what is meant by "immediately following" the observation. If other events occurred, such as driving home, it is conceivable that the researcher may have rehearsed what would be entered in the notes and unconsciously altered the observations or comments. A better plan might have been to carry a small notebook to jot down events or statements made by patients during each observation.

Crootof reread the field notes at the end of each 4 hours of observation. She handled the concept of theoretical saturation by not recording redundant information once a category had been evolved. Such an approach seems logical and appropriate. Review of the field notes at specified times and their referencing according to categorical themes seemed to indicate that sufficient evidence had been collected.

The validation procedures of the study could have been improved greatly by having another researcher read the field notes and identify categories and by checking out the interpretations that Crootof gleaned from the data with the patients. Crootof seems to have validated her observations with patient comments, which is desirable, but could have used additional validation methods.

The categories that emerged from the data appear to be appropriate and to reflect accurately the data that were collected. However, the categories are all in the realm of feelings, and one wonders whether the data may contain other types of categories that are in the realms of physical care, activities performed by patients, and physiologic adaptations. Without reading the entire set of field notes, it would be impossible to suggest other categories that might have emerged from the data.

▧ TEST QUESTIONS AND ANSWERS

Multiple Choice

1. The analysis style that is sometimes referred to as manifest content analysis is:
   - *a. Quasi-statistical style
   - b. Template analysis style
   - c. Editing analysis style
   - d. Immersion/crystallization style

2. The researcher acts as an interpreter who reads through data and develops a categorization scheme on the basis of meaningful segments is the analysis style referred to as:
   - a. Quasi-statistical style
   - b. Template analysis style
   - *c. Editing analysis style
   - d. Immersion/crystallization style

3. Which of the following is *not* a process that plays a role in qualitative analysis:
   - a. Comprehending
   - *b. Attributing
   - c. Synthesizing
   - d. Theorizing

4. The first major step that a researcher must undertake in a qualitative analysis is:
  a. A search for major themes
  b. Entering information into files
  c. The use of quasi-statistics
  *d. Developing a system for organizing and indexing the data

5. Before the advent of computer programs, the main procedure for managing qualitative data was the development of:
  *a. Conceptual files
  b. Core categories
  c. Memos
  d. Themes

6. The process referred to as *constant comparison* involves:
  a. Comparing two researchers' interpretation of the data
  b. Comparing the researchers' interpretation of the data against study participants' interpretation
  *c. Comparing data segments against other segments for similarity and dissimilarity
  d. Comparing data from one study with data from other similar studies

7. Steps generally employed in the analysis of qualitative data include all of the following *except*:
  *a. Testing hypotheses
  b. Searching for themes
  c. Validating themes
  d. Developing a coding scheme

8. Quasi-statistics is essentially a method of:
  a. Statistical analysis
  *b. Validation
  c. Thematic generation
  d. Analytic induction

9. The initial process of breaking down, categorizing, and coding the data is often referred to as:
  a. Axial coding
  b. Core coding
  *c. Open coding
  d. Selective coding

10. Level III coding is sometimes referred to as
  a. Axial coding
  b. Core coding
  c. Open coding
  *d. Selective coding

True/False

(F) 1. One of the features of qualitative analysis is that there are a number of universal formal rules that facilitate the process.

(T) 2. The continuum of qualitative analysis styles ranges from a systematic, standardized style (quasi-statistical) to an intuitive and interpretive style (immersion/crystallization).

(T) 3. The process of *comprehending* is completed when data saturation is achieved.

(F)   4. The process of *recontextualization* involves a sifting of the data and putting pieces together.

(F)   5. Coding schemes are generally developed after the completion of a thematic analysis.

(F)   6. When a computer is used for qualitative analysis, the computer actually performs the coding function.

(T)   7. Like quantitative analysts, qualitative analysts often search for relationships and patterns within the data.

(T)   8. Quasi-statistics involves an accounting of the frequency with which themes are and are not supported by qualitative data.

(F)   9. The grounded theory approach is applied to qualitative data after they have been gathered in the field.

(T)   10. Analytic induction is a method involving an iterative approach to testing hypotheses with qualitative data.

Critical Appraisal and Utilization of Nursing Research

PART VI

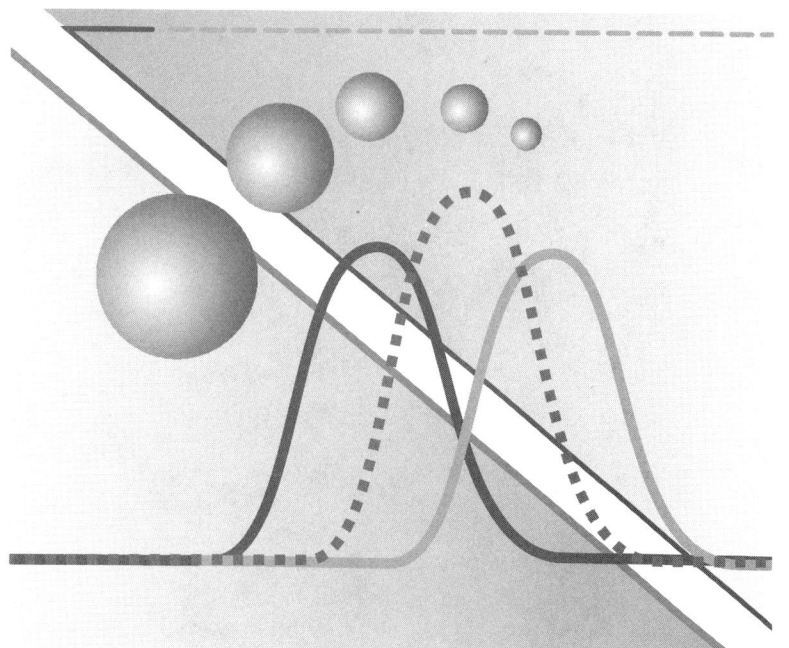

Chapter 13
Critiquing Research Reports

◩ STATEMENT OF INTENT

The major purpose of Chapter 13 is to provide an overall framework for the preparation of a written research critique. The chapter emphasizes that a critique of a study does not mean an exclusive focus on its flaws but rather a balanced assessment of its strengths and weaknesses. A critique essentially involves appraising the decisions the researcher has made in terms of the research problem itself, the theoretical context, methodologic strategies, handling of ethical concerns, and the manner in which the study is described in the report.

In terms of the study methodology, the major decisions that researchers face are different for qualitative and quantitative studies. In quantitative studies, the four most important decisions that a researcher typically faces concern the research design, the specification of the population and the sampling plan, the data collection plan, and the data analysis strategy. In qualitative studies, the key methodologic decisions concern setting, data sources, study participants, and data quality and data analysis. These key decisions should be critiqued with particular care by reviewers.

One final dimension with which the reviewer must be concerned is the researcher's interpretation of the findings. The chapter offers some guidelines for making sense of findings in qualitative studies and in quantitative studies in which the results support the research hypotheses, fail to support them, are contrary to them, and are mixed.

◩ ANSWERS TO SELECTED STUDY-GUIDE EXERCISES

A.1.
1. b
2. c
3. b
4. d
5. b
6. a
7. d
8. c
9. a
10. a

A.2.

1. b	5. b
2. c	6. a
3. d	7. c
4. b	8. d

B.

1. Accuracy
2. Hypothesis
3. Causation
4. Their data
5. Important (useful)
6. Decisions
7. Strengths, weaknesses (virtues, flaws)
8. Substantive/theoretical
9. Methodologic
10. Ethical
11. Interpretive
12. Stylistic/presentational

D.2. Comments on the Study by Champion and Scott: Champion and Scott (1993) conducted a rigorous and interesting study that examined the effectiveness of an intervention on breast self-examination (BSE) performance. Here are a few comments regarding this research.

- Champion and Scott focused on an important topic that has high relevance for nursing and health-care. Developing strategies relating to health promotion has been an important priority for nurse researchers in the 1990s.
- The study was a structured, experimental, quantitative study that can be described as being on the "applied" end of the applied–basic continuum. Although the findings are also relevant to theory, the researchers were primarily interested in developing an effective strategy to address a specific problem—that is, the failure of many women to practice breast self-examination (BSE) regularly.
- The introduction nicely sets the stage for the study. The authors begin by describing the significance of the issue (breast cancer) in the first paragraph. The second paragraph of the report clearly sets forth the purpose of the study: "The purpose of this study was to test selected belief and/or procedural interventions to increase self-reported BSE frequency and proficiency, observer-rated proficiency, and sensitivity using a probability sample of women 35 years of age and older" (p. 163). The remainder of the introduction provides the reader with information about prior interventions, the limitations of earlier research, and the conceptual model guiding the investigators' intervention and research.
- The investigators used the Health Belief Model (HBM) as their conceptual framework. The HBM was an excellent choice, and it is one that has a long and respected history in research on BSE. The researchers do not just pay lip-service to the HBM: their entire intervention (and their data collection) is rooted in the components of the model. Specifically, a major component of the intervention involved strategies to change women's beliefs about the

seriousness of breast cancer, perceived susceptibility to breast cancer, perceived benefits of BSE, and perceived barriers to practicing BSE. In recognition of the fact that women's beliefs and perceptions are different at the outset, the researchers established an *individualized* intervention that took into account initial beliefs.

- The authors specify two hypotheses regarding expected behavioral changes after the intervention. The researchers hypothesized (a) differences between those receiving and those not receiving an intervention; and (b) differences between those receiving both belief and procedural interventions and those receiving only one type of intervention. Both hypotheses concern final outcome measures, that is, changes in the frequency, proficiency, and sensitivity of BSE practice. The authors could have also stated hypotheses concerning expected changes in beliefs after the intervention. (Hypothesis tests relating to changes in beliefs from preintervention to postintervention were, in fact, conducted and therefore implied.)
- The research can be described as evaluation research: the researchers were evaluating the effectiveness of methods to promote BSE. Of the various types of evaluation research, the study could best be described as an impact analysis.
- Commendably, the authors chose a true experimental design to test the effectiveness of the interventions, thus resulting in a study design with strong internal validity. Through randomization, the authors were able to have confidence that the groups would be comparable at the outset with respect to BSE beliefs and practices.
- The design is described as a 2×2 factorial design, which can be diagrammed as follows:

	Procedural Intervention	No Procedural Intervention
Belief Intervention		
No Belief Intervention		

- Although the preceding diagram is an accurate depiction of the manner in which subjects were randomly assigned to groups and the intervention was administered, it appears that the data were not analyzed in this fashion. Rather, a 1×4 strategy, diagrammed as follows, appears to have been used:

Procedural/Belief Intervention	Procedural Intervention	Belief Intervention	No Intervention (Control)

This alternative approach probably simplified the analysis and made the results easier to communicate (*i.e.,* the researchers did not have to worry about an interaction term for groups, and complex interaction terms when groups and the time dimension were considered together).

- Although the research design was an extremely rigorous one, there are some features of the overall design that could have reduced its power. It was noted in Chapter 7 that a powerful design involves maximizing differences between groups. Because the researchers were interested in testing an individualized approach to changing women's beliefs about BSE, they decided to target belief-oriented interventions only on women who scored at or below the midpoint on the baseline belief scales. In other words, the belief interventions consisted of counseling individuals about their beliefs when their beliefs were not consistent, according to the HBM theory, with desired behavior. Thus, women who had above-average beliefs (*i.e.,* believed strongly in the seriousness of breast cancer) did not get the relevant intervention (*i.e.,* the intervention designed to inform women of the seriousness of breast cancer)—even if they were in the Belief Group or in the Procedural/Belief Group. For these women, then, the condition was analogous to those in the control group. Although this approach was consistent with the researchers' desire to have an individualized intervention, the result, methodologically, is that the treatment conditions were not as distinct as they might have been if *all* women in the Belief and Procedural/Belief Groups had been counseled regarding BSE beliefs. (It could be argued that the women who scored below-average on the belief scales needed to have their beliefs *changed*, whereas those with above-average scores needed to have their beliefs *reinforced.*)
- One truly outstanding feature of the researchers' design is their decision to use a long-term follow-up period. The women were assessed with respect to BSE practices 1 year after receiving the intervention (and, although this is not explicitly stated, it seems likely that the sample will be followed again, given the statement on page 164 that women were asked to participate in a 2½-year study). Many BSE studies do a short-term follow-up, making it impossible to draw conclusions about ongoing behavioral changes.
- The researchers adopted an excellent method of sampling. They used random-digit dialing to recruit subjects—a procedure that undoubtedly resulted in a more diverse and representative sample than could have been

achieved by recruiting subjects through clinics or health-care practices. Although a few women in the targeted area (approximately 5%) did not have telephones, this is a relatively small segment of the population to have lost. The researchers also were persistent in attempting to reach a potential subject—they called people who were not home up to 10 times.

- Although the report does not indicate this explicitly, it seems safe to assume that the research team had to place several thousands of calls to recruit the final sample—a very time-consuming but ultimately effective approach. The report stated that 33% of the *eligible* women agreed to participate, meaning that the researchers were able to identify approximately 1000 eligible women through the random calls. However, many calls undoubtedly were made to households that did not have an eligible person (a woman, over age 35, who had no history of breast cancer), and many additional calls must have been made that resulted in busy signals, answering machines, no answers, and hang-ups.

- The researchers were able to recruit 33% of the eligible women who were contacted. Although this is a relatively low percentage in comparison with what would have been ideal (100%), it is actually high when one considers the nature of the commitment the women were being asked to make (participation in a study over a 2½-year period, involving at least two in-home visits).

- It would have been helpful if the researchers had been able to obtain demographic information about eligible women who had refused to participate in the study (*e.g.,* their age, education, race/ethnicity, and so on), so that the nature and extent of response bias could have been analyzed directly. However, the researchers were able to determine that the women participating in their study were fairly similar to the general target population. This information strengthens the readers' confidence that the generalizability of the findings are not severely constrained.

- The researchers were successful in retaining an astonishingly high percentage (94%) of the women who originally completed the first two phases of data collection. The research team must have implemented some excellent contact procedures—and they must also have used well-trained, persuasive, and persistent assistants for scheduling the follow-up visits.

- The final sample for this study was 301 women—a sample that is substantially larger than that used in many studies. The report does not state that a power analysis was performed to determine needed sample size (although this does not mean that a power analysis was *not* performed). Given the many significant findings, it does appear that the sample size was generally adequate. However, the possibility remains that nonsignificant results reflect inadequate power (*i.e.,* Type II errors).

- There is little information in the research report regarding human subjects issues (*i.e.,* privacy and confidentiality, Institutional Review Board approval, and so forth), but this probably reflects space constraints and not the absence of appropriate procedures. The report does indicate that women voluntarily agreed to participate, and that they all signed consent forms. The use of a $25 subject stipend seems appropriate (*i.e.*, noncoercive), given the amount of time the subjects were expected to spend with the researchers.

- The measures used in this study appear to be excellent. The authors were able to document evidence of the validity and reliability of all measures. Moreover, the researchers recognized that one of the limitations of earlier research on BSE interventions was reliance on self-reported frequency and proficiency. They devised a method to *observe* proficiency and sensitivity (lump detection).

- Their analysis plan seemed generally strong. Their analyses included *t*-test, ANOVAs, planned comparisons (not covered in our textbook), and repeated measures MANOVA. It is possible that the analyses would have yielded more sensitive tests if the researchers had controlled for additional covariates (*e.g.*, in the MANOVA with self-reported BSE frequency and proficiency as the dependent variables, preintervention beliefs or demographic characteristics could have been used as covariates to improve the sensitivity of the test of main effects). It is also not clear why the HBM scales were not analyzed in a fashion analogous to the BSE data (using MANOVA or another multivariate procedure) rather than *t*-tests.

- Tables were used effectively to communicate extensive statistical information. The results section did not, however, present a table with means and SDs for the HBM scales (*i.e.*, a table analogous to Table 2 for the BSE measures)—again, perhaps to save on space.

- Given the widespread use of self-reported proficiency data, and the use of both self-reports and observations of proficiency in this study, the researchers would have made an important methodologic contribution by examining the correlation between these two types of measures. Such an analysis is perhaps being handled in a separate research report. (Many other supplementary analyses also seem possible; for example, the researchers could examine the characteristics of women who did and did not alter their BSE behaviors).

- The results of the study were mixed—some findings were consistent with the researchers' hypotheses, and others were not. This is the most common outcome of empirical studies. The researchers generally did an excellent job of interpreting these findings, giving consideration to a range of methodologic and substantive issues. The researchers also did a nice job of pointing out some of the study's limitations (*e.g.*, regarding the generalizability of the findings). The Discussion section also discusses the implications of the study for nurses and for further research in this area.

D.2. **Selected Comments on the Study by Brown and Powell-Cope:** Brown and Powell-Cope (1991) conducted an interesting and well-done study on family caregiving to AIDS patients. Below are some selected comments on this research.

- The researchers investigated a timely topic with relevance and significance to the whole health care community.

- The study was an in-depth qualitative study designed to describe the *experience* of being a family caregiver to an AIDS patient. (The report suggests, however, that the overall research project is an integrated qualitative-quantitative study; the authors note on page 339 that a triangulation of methods was used and that only findings from the qualitative analyses were included in the report).

- The purpose of the study was presented in the last paragraph of the literature review section, just before the Methods section: "The purpose of this grounded theory study was to explore and describe the experience of family members who were caring for persons with AIDS (PWAs) at home" (p. 339). Although the authors postponed a discussion of the study purpose until the end of the literature review, it is concisely described in the first sentence of the abstract. Moreover, the title of the report communicates a considerable amount of information about the study's aim. As indicated in the statement of purpose, the study was *descriptive* and *exploratory*.

- The literature review appears to describe adequately previous research on the family caregiving role (although the authors do not present a *critical* summary that identifies potential weaknesses in this research). The literature review concludes with a discussion of the absence of information about family caregiving within the context of AIDS, thereby justifying the need for the new study.

- Consistent with the grounded theory approach, the researchers did not develop any *a priori* hypotheses. Rather, their analysis and theory generation was developed on the basis of the study participants' own words. Similarly, there are no operational definitions—the definition of the experience of caregiving was allowed to emerge from those living that experience.

- In a descriptive qualitative study such as this one, it is not especially meaningful to identify independent and dependent variables. In fact, there really is no independent variable—that is, the experiences of the family caregivers (which we can construe as the dependent variables) were not examined *in relation* to anything. For example, the investigator did not compare the caregiving experiences of parents versus lovers; male caregivers versus female caregivers; caregivers shortly after an AIDS diagnosis versus those giving care later in the course of the disease; caregivers of homosexual AIDS patients versus those who contracted AIDS some other way, etc.

- The data were collected exclusively by means of personal, unstructured interviews with family caregivers. These were lengthy, in-depth interviews, guided by the primary question: "What has it been like for you living with and taking care of someone with AIDS?" A topic guide was used to ensure that the interviewers covered the key subtopics of interest to the researchers. (The topics covered in the topic guide were not discussed in the report—probably because of space constraints). Rich and lengthy narrative detail about the caregiving experience was obtained in the course of these interviews, which lasted approximately 4½ hours, on average. Presumably, given the use of a grounded theory approach, the questioning evolved over the course of the interviewing as the researchers used the constant comparison technique to code and analyze their data.

- Ideally, the researchers would also have gathered observational data. That is, the researchers would probably have strengthened their understanding of what the caregivers' experiences were by spending time in the homes of AIDS patients during family caregiving episodes. However, such observation would be very time-consuming and costly—not to mention highly sensitive and possibly intrusive.

- A little more detail about the data collection procedures would have been helpful. For example, the report does not indicate how many interviewers there were, what their backgrounds and qualifications were, and what training they received regarding the conduct of the interviews. The report also does not indicate where the interviews occurred (*e.g.*, in the patients' homes, in the caregivers' homes, in some neutral place, and so forth). These aspects may have relevance to an evaluation of the study because they would influence the participants' candor or comfort in the interview situation.

- The sample for the study consisted of 53 family caregivers of people with AIDS or symptomatic HIV infection. This is a relatively large sample in a qualitative study—it yielded more than 200 hours of interview data that had to be transcribed and analyzed. The participants were recruited from several different sources, which helped to reduce the possibility of biases that could be introduced by relying on a single source of referral. Moreover, the researchers deliberately sought out certain types of respondents to ensure adequate data coverage. Thus, the sampling could be described as purposive (or theoretical): "Theoretical sampling was accomplished by selecting respondents based on the need to collect more data to examine categories and their relationships, and to ensure representativeness in the category" (page 339). The sample size was determined on a theoretical basis: when saturation occurred, data collection was terminated.

- The characteristics of the study participants were carefully described in the research report, to help readers understand the nature of the sample. Moreover, the authors note that the AIDS patients being cared for by these caregivers reflected "the demographics of AIDS in the geographical area where the study was conducted" (page 339).

- The report notes that several procedures were undertaken to safeguard the rights of the subjects. The recruitment strategy suggests that participation was purely voluntary, and the report indicates that informed consent was obtained. The procedures for data collection suggest that a situation of "minimal risk" existed. The report notes that all data were treated confidentially, and—despite the inclusion of many excerpts in the text of the report—the privacy of the respondents appears to have been adequately protected. (There is no indication that the study protocols were reviewed by an IRB, but this does not mean that a review did not occur).

- The researchers carefully undertook a number of activities to enhance the trustworthiness of their data. This included member checks, prolonged engagement in the field, method triangulation, and investigator triangulation. Additionally, the researchers organized several focus groups to review and discuss the emerging findings. Focus group members included sample members, caregivers who had not participated in the study, and professionals and community volunteers working in the area of AIDS family caregiving. The report suggests that these focus group discussions helped to improve the validity of the analyses, Because modifications of the theoretical presentation were made on the basis of the feedback from focus group members. The various techniques used in this research were useful in enhancing the confirmability, dependability, and credibility of the data.

- Grounded theory methodology was used to code and analyze the transcribed interview data. The overall goal of the research was to develop a theory of AIDS family caregiving grounded in the empirical data provided by the those giving care. The report provides a good summary of the coding strategies used: "Constant comparative analysis was used as an ongoing technique that included deriving first level codes, or in vivo codes, comparing codes to one another, deriving conceptual categories, and relating categories. Coding strategies included open coding (unrestricted selection of codes from the search for words or phrases that capture the meaning in the transcripts), axial coding (comparison between codes), and selective coding (utilization of frequently occurring codes to create core categories)" (page 339).

- The report does not specifically discuss whether the researchers undertook a systematic search for negative cases in the development of their theory (*i.e.,* situations that did not fit the theory). Such an undertaking is usually an excellent validation procedure. Of course, the failure of the report to mention this activity does not mean that the researchers did not do it.

- In developing their theoretical formulation, the authors took into consideration the broader social context of the study. This context and the investigators' underlying assumptions are carefully presented in the report (page 340).

- The product of the researchers' grounded theory study was a "substantive theory of AIDS family caregiving," presented schematically in Figure 1 of the report. Based on their analyses, the investigators concluded that the basic psychological problem facing the caregivers was uncertainty, and that a core task was to make a transition through uncertainty. Uncertainty, according to their analysis, is a multidimensional construct: five subcategories detailing its multiple aspects were identified. For each of these subcategories, the researchers' analyses showed various stages and strategies.

Each subcategory is explained in some detail in the report, and excellent illustrations (excerpts from the interviews) are provided.

■ Although space constraints may have hampered the authors' ability to explicate their findings in greater detail, it would have been interesting to learn something about any systematic variation occurring within the data. Were the patterns of caregiving similar for male and female caregivers? Parents and lovers or spouses? Older and younger caregivers?

■ The Discussion section of the report nicely ties the authors' conceptualization of uncertainty to previous research on this construct, and notes that researchers have primarily studied uncertainty in relation to *patients* rather than caregivers. The discussion section also provides some interesting suggestions for the application of the findings (*i.e.*, the development of clinical therapeutics in the form of anticipatory guidance) and for further research in this area. Although the authors did not specifically recommend this, a replication in the current social context (when there is less stigma and ignorance about AIDS and perhaps less uncertainty about it as well) would be desirable to examine whether the researcher's theoretical formulation is still relevant.

▧ TEST QUESTIONS AND ANSWERS

Multiple Choice

1. The major purpose of a research critique is to assess:
   - a. The strengths of a research study
   - b. The limitations of a research study
   - *c. Both of the above
   - d. Neither of the above

2. A research critique should be a(n):
   - a. Criticism of a researcher's faulty methodologic decisions
   - b. Inventory of needed improvements in research design
   - c. Analysis of a study's internal validity problems
   - *d. Balanced appraisal of a study's strengths and weaknesses

3. If a reader concluded that a quantitative study had internal validity problems, this would involve a critique of which of the following dimensions of the study?
   - a. Substantive
   - *b. Methodologic
   - c. Ethical
   - d. Interpretive

4. The reviewer's concern about the study's relevance to nursing would be focusing on which dimension?
   - *a. Substantive
   - b. Methodologic
   - c. Ethical
   - d. Stylistic

5. The handling of response set biases concerns which of the following methodologic decisions in a quantitative study?

a. Research design

b. Sampling plan

*c. Data collection procedures

d. Data analysis plan

6. The researcher's decision to randomly assign research subjects concerns which of the following methodologic decisions?

*a. Research design

b. Sampling plan

c. Study population

d. Data collection plan

7. A qualitative researcher's decision to conduct participant observation concerns which of the following methodologic decisions?

a. Setting

b. Data sources

c. Sampling

d. Data quality/analysis

8. If a reviewer perceived that the researcher failed to consider important study weaknesses in the concluding section of the report, this would involve a critique of which of the following dimensions?

a. Substantive

b. Methodologic

c. Ethical

*d. Interpretive

9. Which of the following interpretations is acceptable as worded?

a. The study proved that cigarette smoking causes lung cancer

b. This study indicated that there is no relationship between use of an IUD and PID

*c. The findings suggest that cholesterol influences heart function

d. The results demonstrate that lithium has hazardous side effects

10. Suppose a quantitative researcher hypothesized that a relationship existed between nurses' leadership behavior and job satisfaction. Correlational analysis revealed an r of .60 that had a p value beyond the .001 level. The researcher may conclude all the following *except*:

a. The greater the leadership behavior of the nurse, the higher the degree of job satisfaction

b. The data analysis suggested that the research hypothesis was correct

c. A statistically significant relationship existed between nurses' leadership behaviors and job satisfaction

*d. High levels of leadership behavior caused high job satisfaction

11. Nonsignificant statistical findings indicate that the null hypothesis is:

*a. Retained

b. Rejected

c. Proved

d. Inconclusive

12. The person who critiques a published research report should strive to:

a. Withhold overly critical comments that would discourage the researcher

b. Focus primarily on the data analysis and findings

c. Judge the merits of the study based on the researcher's background

*d. Remain as objective and balanced as possible

True/False

(F)   1. Only researchers can adequately evaluate the decisions that another researcher makes in conducting a study.

(F)   2. Publication of a research report indicates that the study was of high quality.

(F)   3. The more faulty decisions a reviewer can identify, the more rigorous the critique is.

(T)   4. Most research studies have inadequacies as well as adequacies.

(T)   5. Critical appraisals of research reports play an important role in the advancement of knowledge.

(F)   6. The major focus of a research critique is the evaluation of the analyses and results.

(T)   7. Interpretation of results in quantitative studies refers to the process of attaching meaning to the numeric values obtained in statistical testing.

(F)   8. The term *mixed results* refers to the condition in which some of the researcher's results conflict with the results of prior studies and others do not.

(T)   9. A statistically significant result may not have any practical value.

(F) 10. When all the research hypotheses have been supported, it is acceptable practice for the researcher to infer causality.

(F) 11. Statistically significant correlations demonstrate a causal relationship.

(T) 12. A statistically nonsignificant result may nevertheless have practical value.

Chapter 14
Utilization of Nursing Research

▨ STATEMENT OF INTENT

The purpose of this chapter is to sensitize nursing students to the need for increased utilization of findings from nursing research investigations. Although research utilization is often beyond the control of individual clinical nurses, the entire nursing community has a role to play in making sure that nursing practice is built on as solid a foundation as possible. This chapter describes both the potential for utilizing research findings and the current status of utilization—descriptions that illuminate the current gap between knowledge production and knowledge utilization. The chapter discusses what some of the barriers to research utilization are and also provides some suggested strategies for overcoming those barriers. A concluding section of the chapter discusses the steps that need to be undertaken to evaluate the utilization potential of a research finding and to implement a utilization project.

▨ COMMENTS ON THE ACTUAL RESEARCH EXAMPLE IN THE TEXTBOOK

The report by Kilpack and colleagues (1991) was an interesting description of a utilization project. Below are a few comments on the study.

- This is an excellent example of a project undertaken by a team of clinical nurses in direct response to a clinical problem. The team undertook a full-blown, successful utilization project that involved many staff within the hospital. It appears that staff cooperation was high and organizational support was strong.
- The team adopted the problem identification model of utilization. They started with a problematic situation, reviewed and assessed the research literature, developed an implementation plan, and then evaluated the outcomes resulting from the implementation. (Although the report does not describe in detail the assessment of implementation potential, we must assume that this was successfully undertaken or the team would not have proceeded to the next step.)
- The report concluded with six specific recommendations, which the hospital implemented on the basis of the project. Other hospitals with a similar

problem of a high rate of inpatient falls could also implement many of these recommendations.

■ The study illustrates that practicing nurses, even in a relatively small hospital, can profitably undertake a utilization project. It appears that members of the hospital staff conducted the project without any outside assistance.

■ Despite the excellence of this project, the team might have profited from collaboration with a researcher, who might have offered suggestions for undertaking a more sophisticated analysis of their data.

◤ ANSWERS TO SELECTED STUDY-GUIDE EXERCISES

A.1.

1. b (also c)
2. a
3. c
4. a
5. a (also b and c)

6. b (also a and c)
7. c
8. c
9. b (also c)
10. b (also a and c)

B.

1. Research utilization
2. Gap
3. Conduct and Utilization Research in Nursing (CURN)
4. Western Interstate Commission for Higher Education (WICHE) Regional Program for Nursing Research Development

5. Replicated
6. Implementation potential
7. Transferability
8. The cost/benefit of *not* implementing it

◤ TEST QUESTIONS AND ANSWERS

Multiple Choice

1. If a specific nursing procedure in a hospital were modified on the basis of research findings, this would be an example of:

   a. Persuasion stage of adoption
   b. Awareness stage of adoption
   *c. Instrumental utilization
   d. Conceptual utilization

2. The awareness stage of adoption is similar to:

   *a. Conceptual utilization
   b. Instrumental utilization
   c. Decision accretion
   d. None of the above

3. Utilization projects such as the WICHE and the CURN projects showed that research utilization is impeded by:

*a. The shortage of reliable, scientifically sound nursing studies with clear clinical implications

b. The shortage of publication outlets for nurse researchers

c. The long time lag between completion of a study and the appearance of the research report in nursing journals

d. Lack of support for research and utilization from the federal government

4. Which of the following is *not* a major barrier to research utilization in nursing?

a. The failure of many nurses to be academically prepared to critically evaluate nursing research studies

b. The failure of hospital and other organizations that employ nurses to reward nurses who engage in utilization efforts

c. The failure of nurse researchers to replicate studies that show promise for utilization

*d. The failure of nurse researchers to engage in any clinically relevant studies

5. Researchers can improve the prospects for utilization by doing all of the following *except*:

a. Conducting high-quality, scientifically sound studies

b. Disseminating results to a broad audience

*c. Offering clinical nurses resource support for a utilization project

d. Discussing the clinical implications of their study results in their research reports

6. Which of the following strategies for utilization is most amenable to adoption by nursing students?

a. Preparing integrative reviews

b. Replicating research studies

c. Making presentations at nursing conferences

*d. Reading professional journals widely and critically

7. An assessment of the implementation potential of a nursing innovation includes which of the following activities?

a. Assessment of clinical relevance

*b. Cost/benefit assessment

c. Assessment of the study's generalizability

d. Assessment of the scientific merit of the study

8. If an innovation reported in the research literature is judged not to be clinically relevant, the next step would be to:

*a. Search for another topic in the research literature

b. Evaluate the scientific merit of the studies in which the innovation was tested

c. Assess the transferability of the findings to a new setting

d. Determine the costs and benefits of implementing the innovation

True/False

(T)   1. Conceptual utilization of research involves a situation in which individuals are influenced in their thinking about an issue based on their knowledge of a study.

(F)   2. Decision accretion occurs when a nurse decides to implement the findings from a rigorous research investigation.

(F)   3. Studies have generally found that nurses have failed to utilize research findings at any point along the utilization continuum.

(T)   4. The persuasion stage of adoption refers to a situation in which consumers are aware of a research finding and believe that it ought to result in changes.

(F)   5. A well-known nursing research utilization project is the American Nurses' Association Project on the Standards of Nursing Practice.

(T)   6. Communication problems between nurse researchers and clinical nurses are a stumbling block to utilization.

(T)   7. Replication of studies must be a critical part of efforts to increase research utilization.

(F)   8. The three broad classes of criteria for research utilization are clinical relevance, scientific merit, and statistical significance.

(F)   9. Nursing students have a negligible role to play in promoting the utilization of nursing research studies.

(T)   10. An important aspect of assessing the implementation potential of an innovation is evaluating the transferability of the findings to a new setting.

Transparency Masters

PART VII

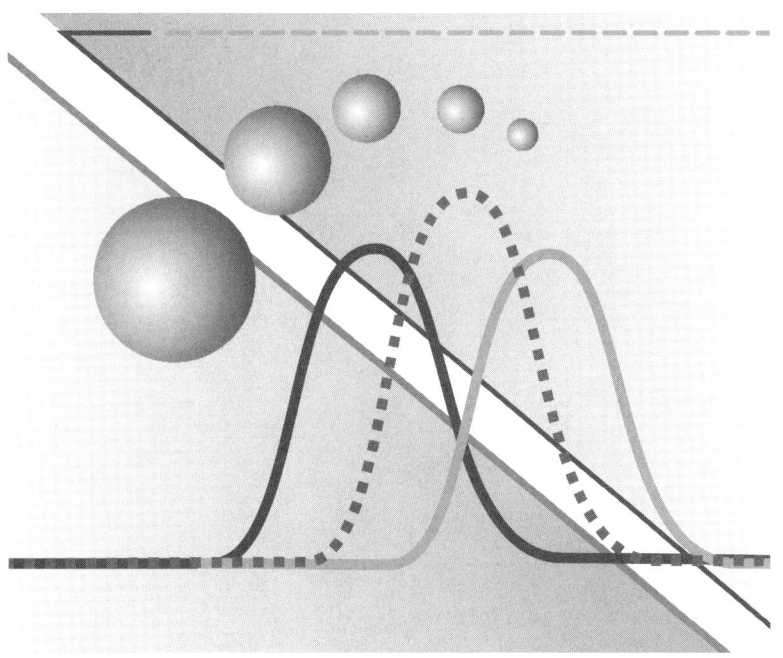

Table 1–1. Major Assumptions of the Positivist and Naturalistic Paradigms

Philosophical Question	Positivist Paradigm Assumptions	Naturalistic Paradigm Assumptions
Ontologic (What is the nature of reality?)	Reality exists; there is a real world driven by real natural causes.	Reality is multiple and subjective, mentally constructed by individuals.
Epistemologic (How is the inquirer related to those being researched?)	Inquirer is independent from those being researched; the findings are not influenced by the researcher.	The inquirer interacts with those being researched; findings are the creation of the interactive process.
Axiologic (What is the role of values in the inquiry?)	Values and biases are to be held in check; objectivity is sought.	Subjectivity and values are inevitable and desirable.
Methodologic (How is knowledge obtained?)	Deductive processes	Inductive processes
	Emphasis on discrete, specific concepts	Emphasis on entirety of some phenomenon, holistic
	Verification of researcher's hunches	Emerging interpretations grounded in participants' experiences
	Fixed design	Flexible design
	Tight controls over context	Context-bound
	Emphasis on measured, quantitative information; statistical analysis	Emphasis on narrative information; qualitative analysis
	Seeks generalizations	Seeks patterns

Table 1–2. Research Purposes and Research Questions

Purpose	Types of Questions: Quantitative Research	Types of Questions: Qualitative Research
Identification		What is this phenomenon? What is its name?
Description	How prevalent is the phenomenon? How often does the phenomenon occur? What are the characteristics of the phenomenon?	What are the dimensions of the phenomenon? What variations exist? What is important about the phenomenon?
Exploration	What factors are related to the phenomenon? What are the antecedents of the phenomenon?	What is the full nature of the phenomenon? What is really going on here? What is the process by which the phenomenon evolves or is experienced?
Explanation	What are the measurable associations between phenomena? What factors caused the phenomenon? Does the theory explain the phenomenon?	How does the phenomenon work? Why does the phenomenon exist? What is the meaning of the phenomenon? How did the phenomenon occur?
Prediction and control	What will happen if we alter a phenomenon or introduce an intervention? If phenomenon X occurs, will phenomenon Y follow? How can we make the phenomenon happen, or alter its nature or prevalence? Can the occurrence of the phenomenon be controlled?	

Table 2–1. Key Terms Used in Quantitative and Qualitative Research

Concept	Quantitative Term	Qualitative Term
Person contributing information	Subject Study participant Respondent	— Study participant Informant
Person undertaking the study	Researcher Investigator Scientist	Researcher Investigator —
That which is being investigated	— Concepts Constructs Variables (independent, dependent)	Phenomena, topics Concepts —
System of organizing concepts	Theory, theoretical framework Conceptual framework, conceptual model	Theory
Information gathered	Data (numerical values)	Data (narrative descriptions)
Connections between concepts	Relationships (cause-and-effect, functional)	Patterns of association

Box 2-1

Example of Quantitative Data

Question: Thinking about the past week, how depressed would you say you
             have been on a scale from 0 to 10, where 0 means "not at all" and
             10 means "the most possible"?

Data: 9   (Subject 1)
             0   (Subject 2)
             4   (Subject 3)

Example of Qualitative Data

Question: Tell me about how you've been feeling lately—have you felt sad or depressed at all, or have you generally been in good spirits?

Data: Well, actually, I've been pretty depressed lately, to tell you the truth. I wake up each morning and I can't seem to think of anything to look forward to. I mope around the house all day, kind of in despair. I just can't seem to shake the blues, and I've begun to think I need to go see a shrink. (Participant 1)

I can't remember ever feeling better in my life. I just got promoted to a new job that makes me feel like I can really get ahead in my company. And I've just gotten engaged to a really great guy who is very special. (Participant 2)

I've had a few ups and downs the past week, but basically things are on a pretty even keel. I don't have too many complaints. (Participant 3)

Table 3-1. Example of Terms Relating to Research Problems

Term	Example
Topic/focus	Side effects in chemotherapy patients
Research problem	Nausea and vomiting are common side effects among chemotherapy patients. What intervention can reduce or prevent these side effects?
Statement of purpose	The purpose of the study is to test an intervention to reduce chemotherapy-induced side effects—specifically, to compare the effectiveness of patient-controlled and nurse-administered antiemetic therapy for controlling nausea and vomiting in chemotherapy patients.
Research question (Problem statement)	What is the relative effectiveness of patient-controlled antiemetic therapy versus nurse-controlled antiemetic therapy with regard to (a) medication consumption and (b) control of nausea and vomiting in chemotherapy patients?
Hypotheses	(1) Subjects receiving antiemetic therapy by way of a patient-controlled pump will report less nausea than subjects receiving the therapy by way of nurse-administration; (2) Subjects receiving antiemetic therapy by way of a patient-controlled pump will vomit less than subjects receiving the therapy by way of nurse-administration; (3) Subjects receiving antiemetic therapy by way of a patient-controlled pump will consume less medication than subjects receiving the therapy by way of nurse-administration.
Aims/objectives	This study seeks to accomplish the following objectives: (1) to develop and implement two alternative procedures for administering antiemetic therapy for patients receiving moderate emetogenic chemotherapy (patient-controlled versus nurse-controlled); (2) to test three hypotheses concerning the relative effectiveness of the alternative procedures on medication consumption and control of side effects; and (3) to use the findings to develop recommendations for possible changes to therapeutic procedures.

Table 3–4. Examples of Simple and Complex Hypotheses

Hypothesis	Independent Variable	Dependent Variable	Simple or Complex
Older patients are more at risk of experiencing a fall than younger patients.	Age of patients	Falling behavior	Simple
Infants born to heroin-addicted mothers have lower birth weights than infants with nonaddicted mothers.	Addiction versus nonaddiction of mother	Birth weight of infant	Simple
Structured preoperative support is more effective in reducing surgical patients' perceptions of pain and requests for analgesics than structured postoperative support.	Timing of nursing intervention	Patients' pain perceptions; requests for analgesics	Complex
Positive health practices are favorably affected by high self-esteem and greater amounts of social support.	Self-esteem; social support	Health practices	Complex

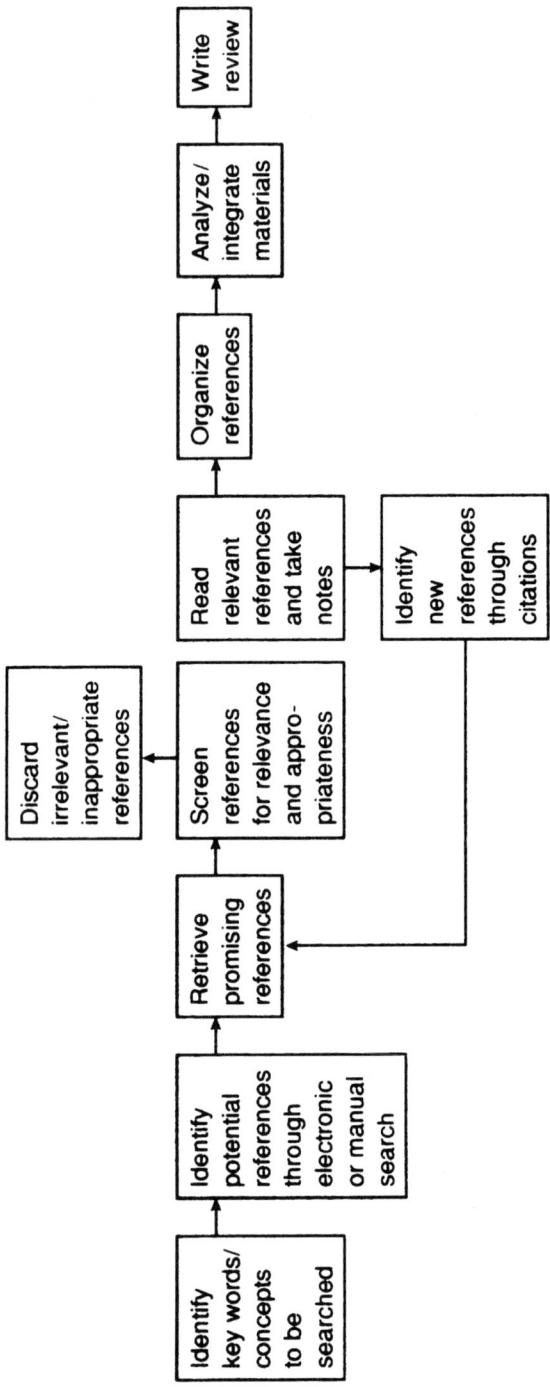

Figure 4–2. Flow of tasks in preparing a written research review.
Copyright © 1997 Lippincott-Raven Publishers
Polit/Hungler: Essentials of Nursing Research, fourth edition

Table 4-1. Examples of Stylistic Difficulties for Research Reviews

Inappropriate Style or Wording	Recommended Change
1. It is known that unmet expectations engender anxiety.	Several experts (Abraham, 1996; Lawrence, 1995) have asserted that unmet expectations engender anxiety.
2. The woman who does not participate in childbirth preparation classes tends to manifest a high degree of stress during labor.	Previous studies have indicated that women who participate in preparation for childbirth classes manifest less stress during labor than those who do not (Klotz, 1996; McTygue, 1995).
3. Studies have proved that doctors and nurses do not fully understand the psychobiologic dynamics of recovery from a myocardial infarction.	The studies by O'Hara (1995) and Carson (1996) suggest that doctors and nurses do not fully understand the psychobiologic dynamics of recovery from a myocardial infarction.
4. Attitudes cannot be changed overnight.	Attitudes have been found to be relatively enduring attributes that cannot be changed overnight (O'Connell, 1995; Valentine, 1996).
5. Responsibility is an intrinsic stressor.	According to Doctor A. Cassard, an authority on stress, responsibility is an intrinsic stressor (Cassard, 1994, 1995).

NOTE: All references are fictitious.

Table 6–1. Dimensions of Quantitative Research Designs

Dimension	Design	Major Features
Control over independent variable	• Experimental	Manipulation of independent variable, control group, randomization
	• Quasi-experimental	Manipulation of independent variable but no randomization or no control group
	• Nonexperimental	No manipulation of independent variable
Type of group comparisons	• Between-subjects	Participants in groups being compared are different people
	• Within-subjects	Participants in groups being compared are the same people
Number of data collection points	• Cross-sectional	Data collected at one point in time
	• Longitudinal	Data collected at multiple points in time over extended period
Occurrence of independent and dependent variable	• Retrospective	Study begins with dependent variable and looks backward for cause or influence
	• Prospective	Study begins with independent variable and looks forward for the effect
Setting	• Naturalistic	Data collected in a real-world setting
	• Laboratory	Data collected in artificial, contrived setting

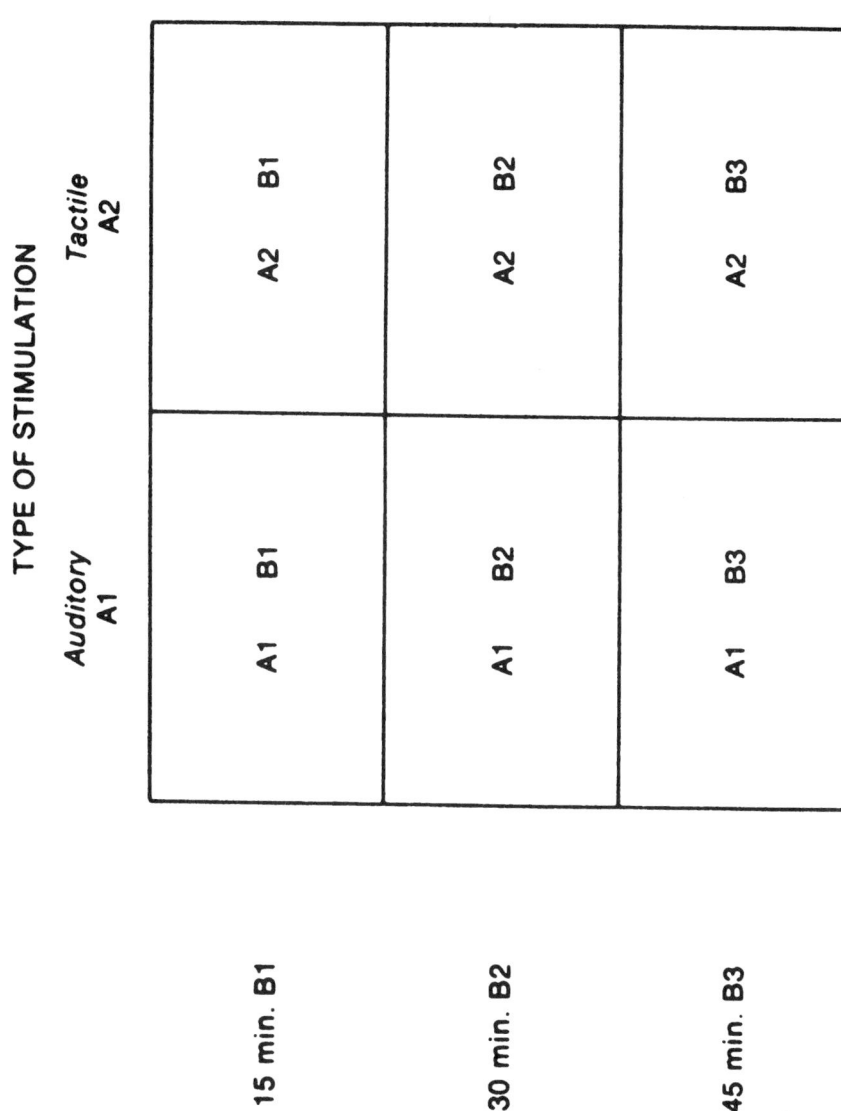

TYPE OF STIMULATION

Auditory A1   Tactile A2

	Auditory A1	Tactile A2
15 min. B1	A1 B1	A2 B1
30 min. B2	A1 B2	A2 B2
45 min. B3	A1 B3	A2 B3

DAILY EXPOSURE

Figure 6–1. Schematic diagram of a factorial experiment.
Copyright © 1997 Lippincott-Raven Publishers
Polit/Hungler: Essentials of Nursing Research, fourth edition

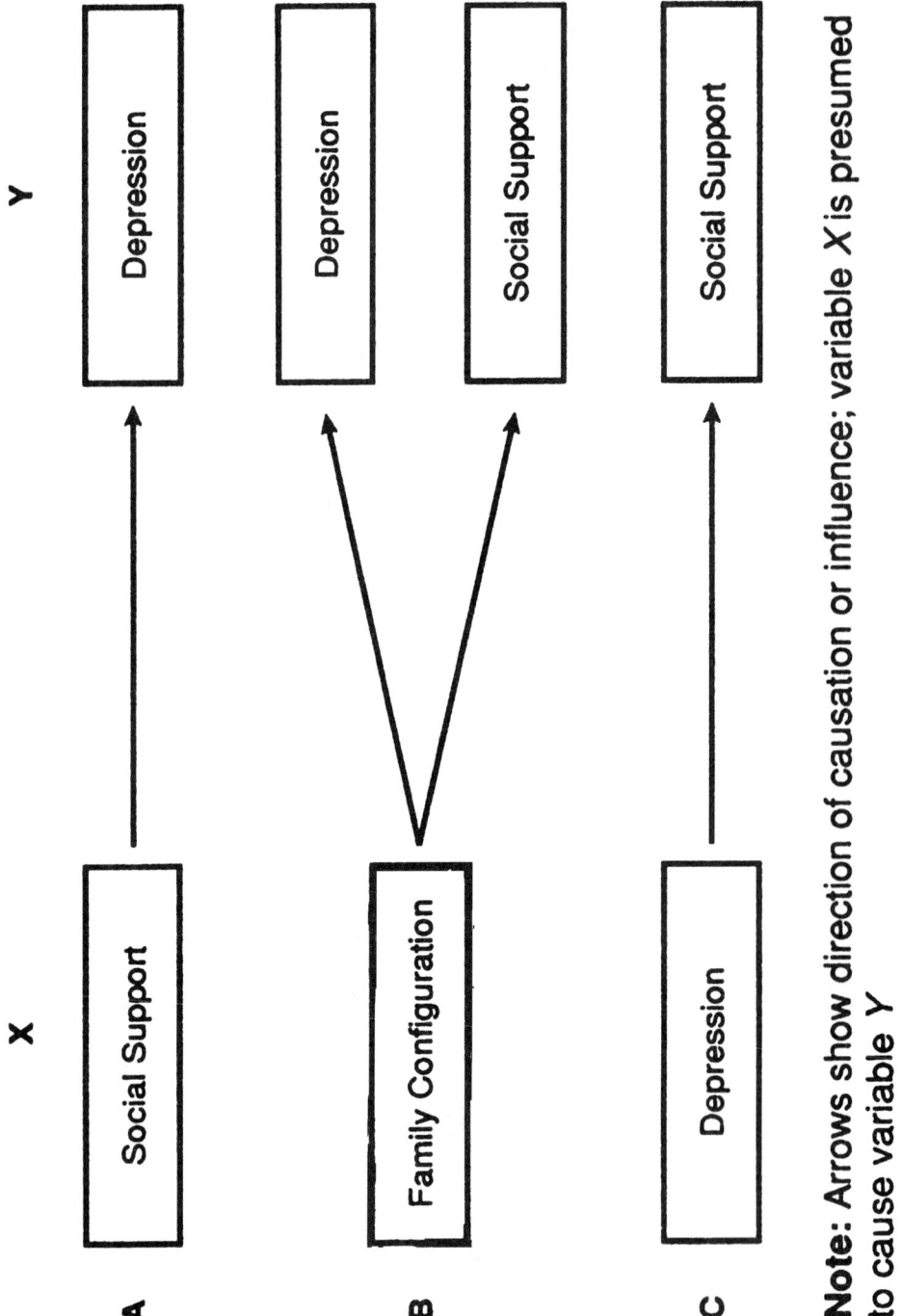

Figure 6–2. Alternative explanations for relationship between depression and social support in cancer patients.

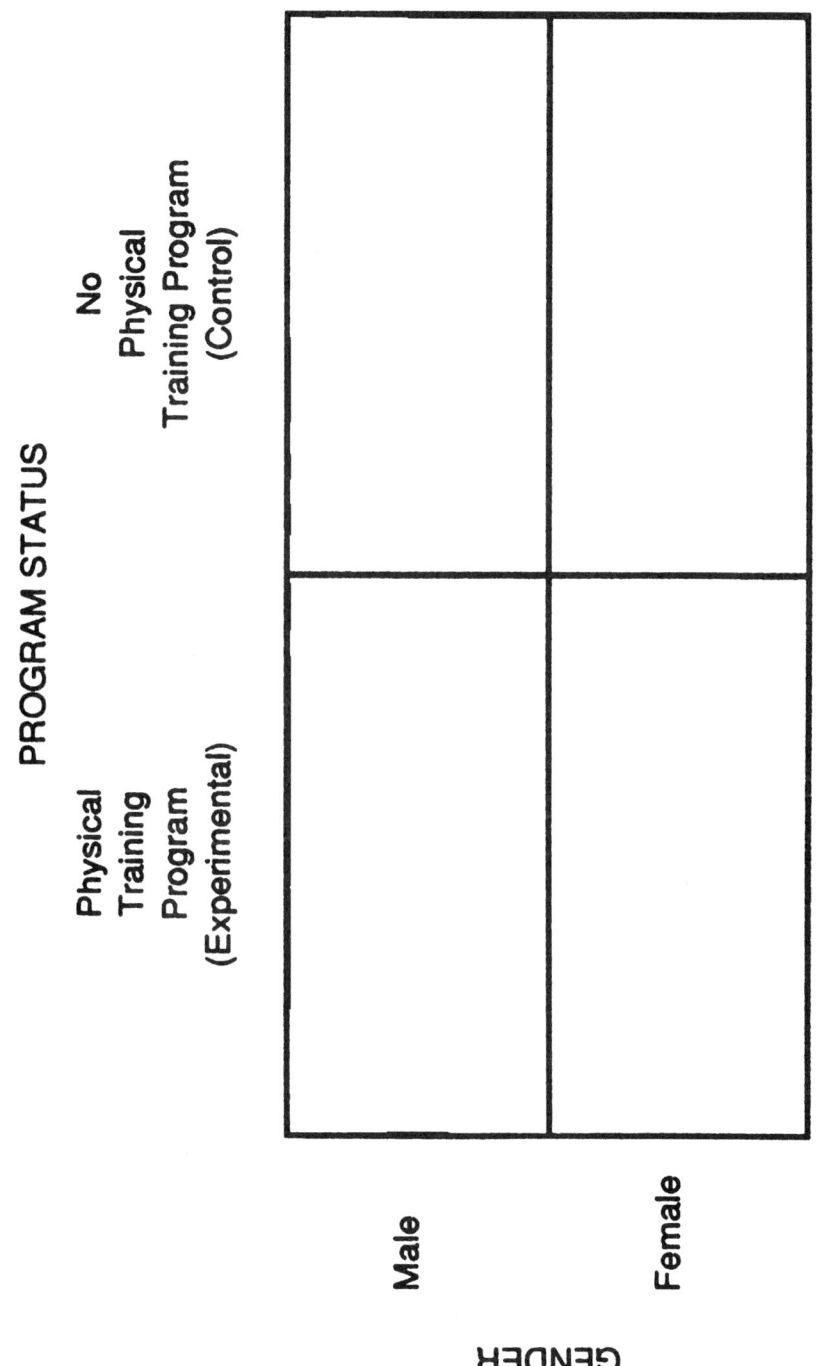

Figure 6–3. Schematic diagram of a randomized block design.

Table 7–1. Overview of Qualitative Research Traditions

Discipline	Research Tradition	Domain of Inquiry
Anthropology	Ethnography	Culture Holistic view of a culture
	Ethnoscience (cognitive anthropology)	Mapping of the cognitive world of a culture; a culture's shared meanings, semantic rules
Psychology/ Philosophy	Phenomenology	Lived Experience Experiences of individuals within their lifeworld
	Hermeneutics	Experiences of individuals as access to sociocultural context
Psychology	Ethology	Behavior and Events Behavior observed over time in natural context
	Ecologic psychology	Behavior as influenced by the environment
Sociology	Grounded theory	Social Settings Social structural processes within a social setting
	Ethnomethodology	Manner by which shared agreement is achieved in social settings
	Symbolic interaction (semiotics)	Manner by which people make sense of social interactions
Sociolinguistics	Discourse analysis	Human Communication Forms and rules of conversation

Table 9–1. Examples of Question Types

Open-Ended

1. What led to your decision to stop using oral contraceptives?
2. What did you do when you discovered you had AIDS?

Closed-Ended

1. Dichotomous Question
   Have you ever been hospitalized?
   ( ) 1. Yes
   ( ) 2. No

2. Multiple-Choice Question
   How important is it to you to avoid a pregnancy at this time?
   ( ) 1. Extremely important
   ( ) 2. Very important
   ( ) 3. Somewhat important
   ( ) 4. Not at all important

3. "Cafeteria" Question
   People have different opinions about the use of estrogen-replacement therapy for women in menopause. Which of the following statements best represents your point of view?
   ( ) 1. Estrogen replacement is dangerous and should be totally banned.
   ( ) 2. Estrogen replacement may have some undesirable side effects that suggest the need for caution in its use.
   ( ) 3. I am undecided about my views on estrogen-replacement therapy.
   ( ) 4. Estrogen replacement has many beneficial effects that merit its promotion.
   ( ) 5. Estrogen replacement is a wonder cure that should be administered routinely to menopausal women.

4. Rank-Order Question
   People value different things about life. Below is a list of principles or ideals that are often cited when people are asked to name things they value most. Please indicate the order of importance of these values to you by placing a *1* beside the most important, *2* beside the next most important, and so forth.
   ( ) Achievement and success
   ·( ) Family relationships
   ( ) Friendships and social interaction
   ( ) Health
   ( ) Money
   ( ) Religion

5. Forced-Choice Question
   Which statement most closely represents your point of view?
   ( ) 1. What happens to me is my own doing.
   ( ) 2. Sometimes, I feel I don't have enough control over my life.

6. Rating Question
   On a scale from 0 to 10, where 0 means extremely dissatisfied and 10 means extremely satisfied, how satisfied are you with the nursing care you received during your hospitalization?

Extremely dissatisfied										Extremely satisfied
0	1	2	3	4	5	6	7	8	9	10

Table 9–2. Example of a Likert Scale to Measure Attitudes Toward the Mentally Ill

Direction of Scoring*		Responses†					Score Person 1 (✓)	Person 2 (X)
		SA	A	?	D	SD		
+	1. People who have had a mental illness can become normal, productive citizens after treatment.		✓			X	4	1
−	2. People who have been patients in mental hospitals should not be allowed to have children.			X		✓	5	3
−	3. The best way to handle patients in mental hospitals is to restrict their activity as much as possible.		X		✓		4	2
+	4. Many patients in mental hospitals develop normal, healthy relationships with staff members and other patients.			✓	X		3	2
+	5. There should be an expanded effort to get the mentally ill out of institutional settings and back into their communities.	✓				X	5	1
−	6. Because the mentally ill cannot be trusted, they should be kept under constant guard.		X			✓	5	2
	TOTAL SCORE						26	11

*Researchers would not indicate the direction of scoring on a Likert scale administered to subjects. The scoring direction is indicated in this table for illustrative purposes only.
†SA, strongly agree; A, agree: ?, uncertain; D, disagree; SD, strongly disagree.

NURSE PRACTITIONERS

competent	7*	6	5	4	3	2	1	incompetent
worthless	1	2	3	4	5	6	7	valuable
important								unimportant
pleasant								unpleasant
bad								good
cold								warm
responsible								irresponsible
successful								unsuccessful

*The score values would not be printed on the form administered to actual subjects. The numbers are presented here solely for the purpose of illustrating how semantic differentials are scored.

Figure 9–1. Example of a semantic differential

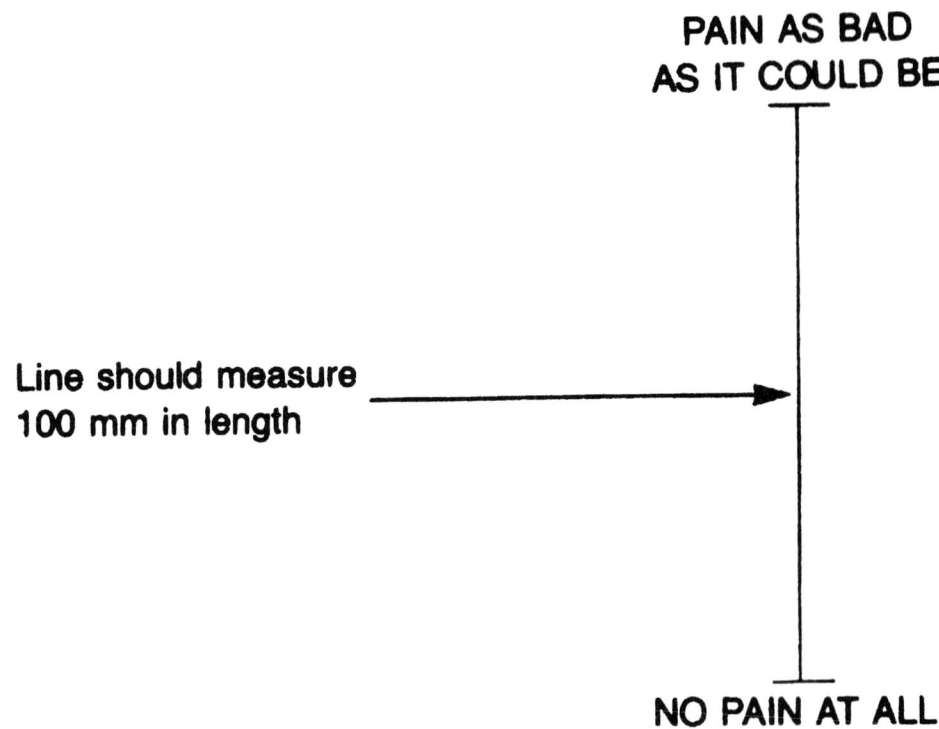

Figure 9–2. Example of a visual analog scale

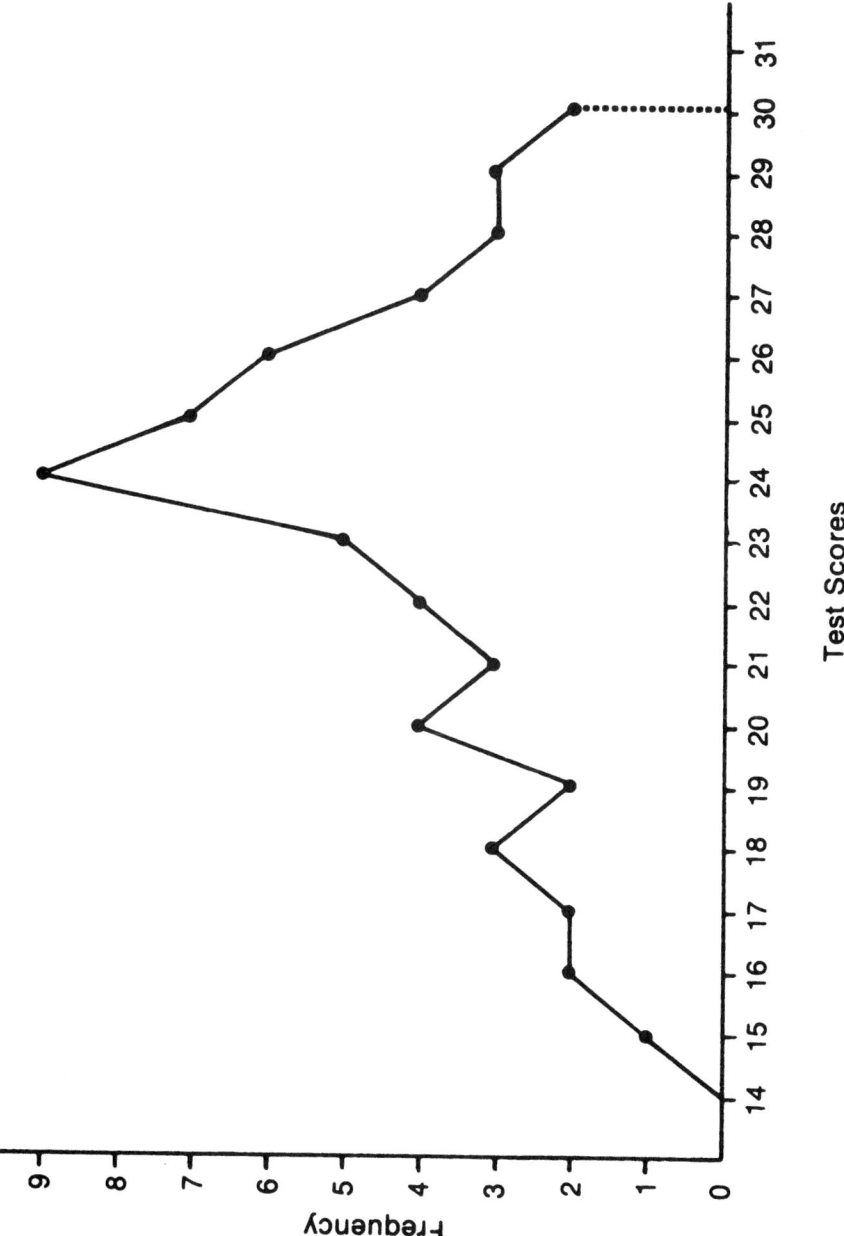

Figure 11–1. Frequency polygon of test scores
Copyright © 1997 Lippincott-Raven Publishers
Polit/Hungler: Essentials of Nursing Research, fourth edition

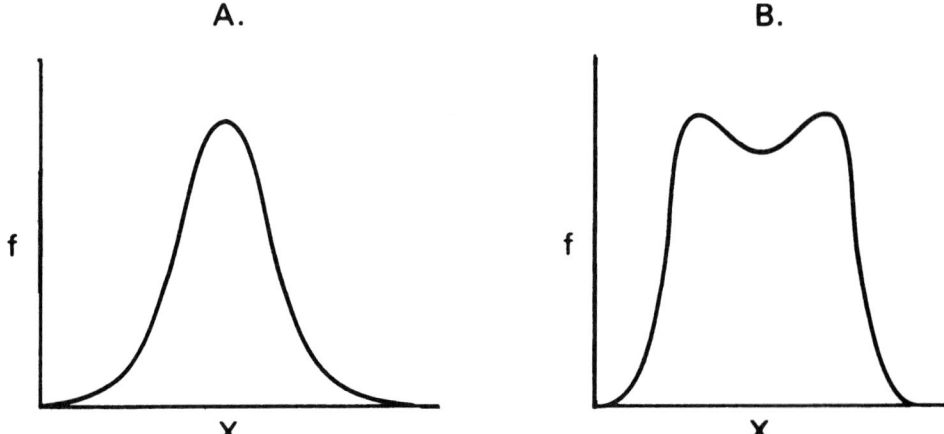

Figure 11–2. Examples of symmetric distributions

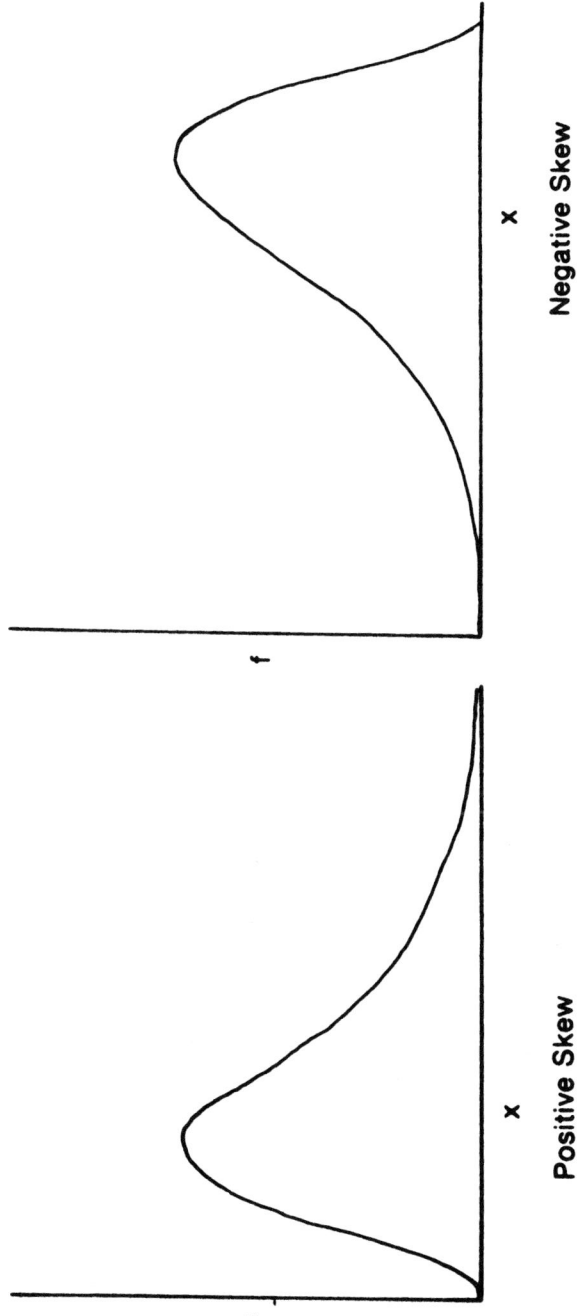

Figure 11–3. Examples of skewed distributions
Copyright © 1997 Lippincott-Raven Publishers
Polit/Hungler: Essentials of Nursing Research, fourth edition

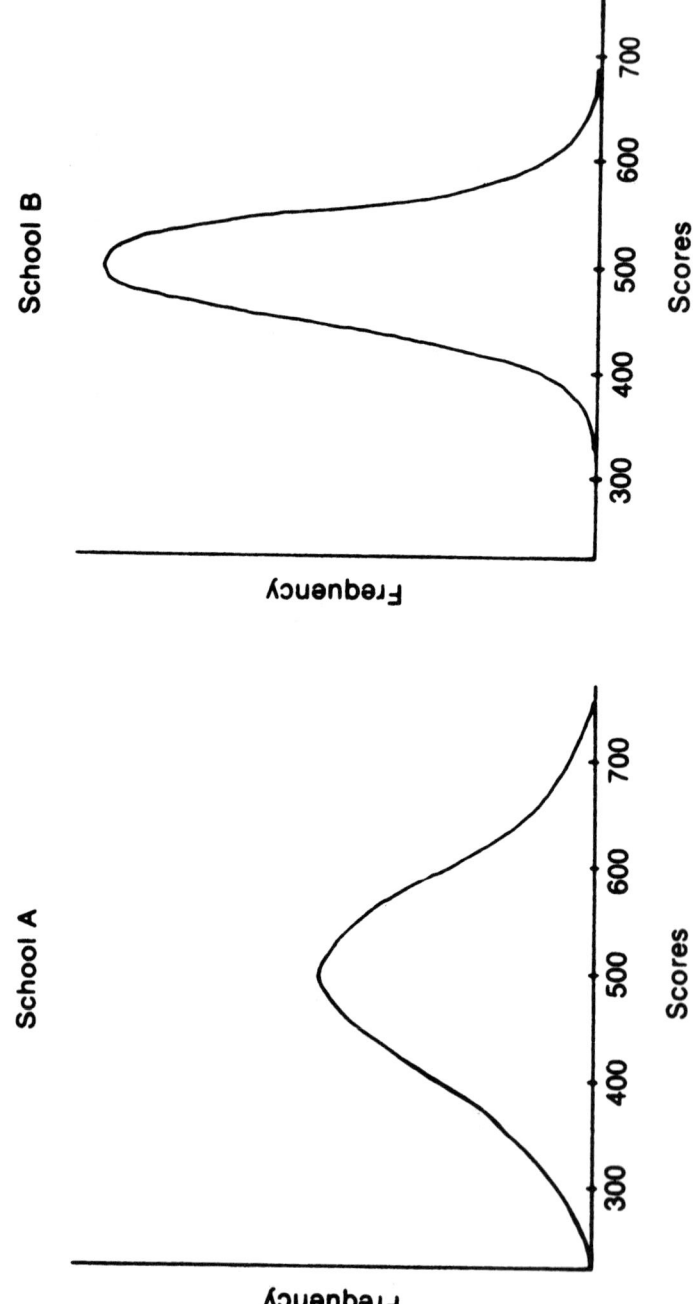

Figure 11–4. Two distributions of different variability
Copyright © 1997 Lippincott-Raven Publishers
Polit/Hungler: Essentials of Nursing Research, fourth edition

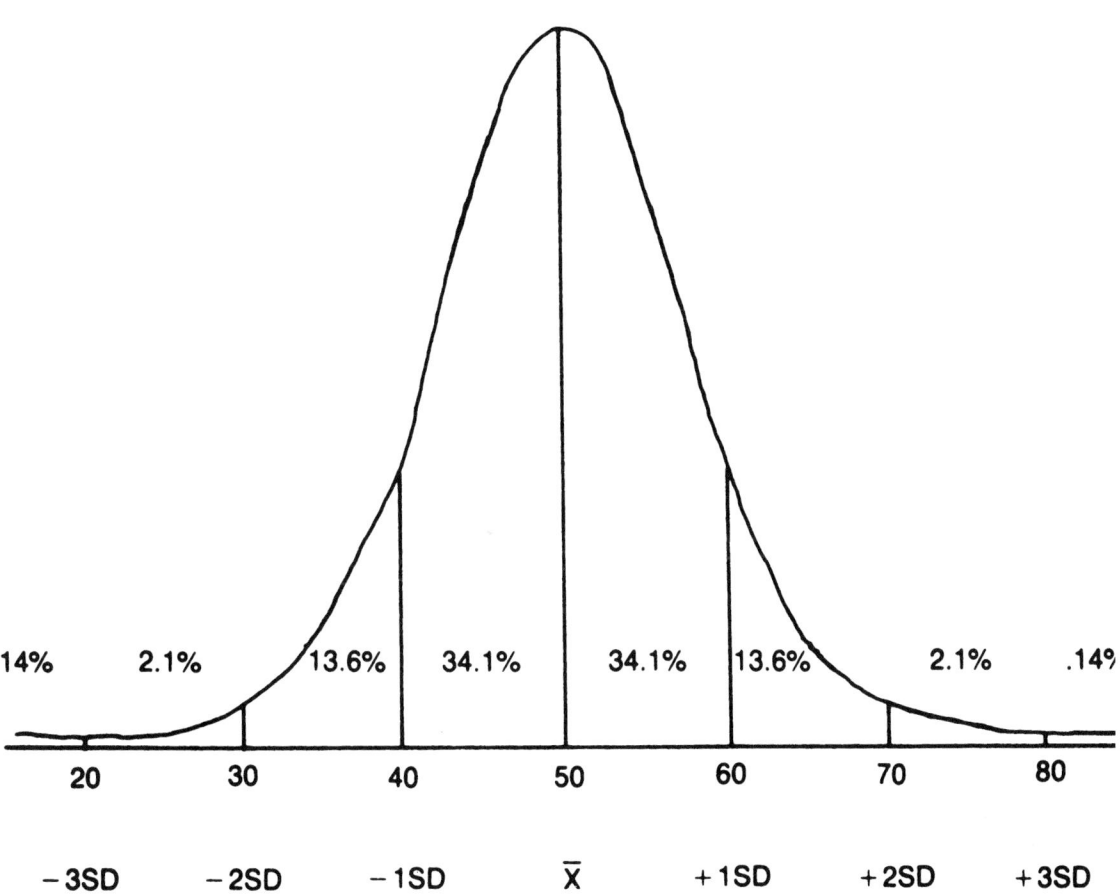

Figure 11–5. Standard deviations in a normal distribution

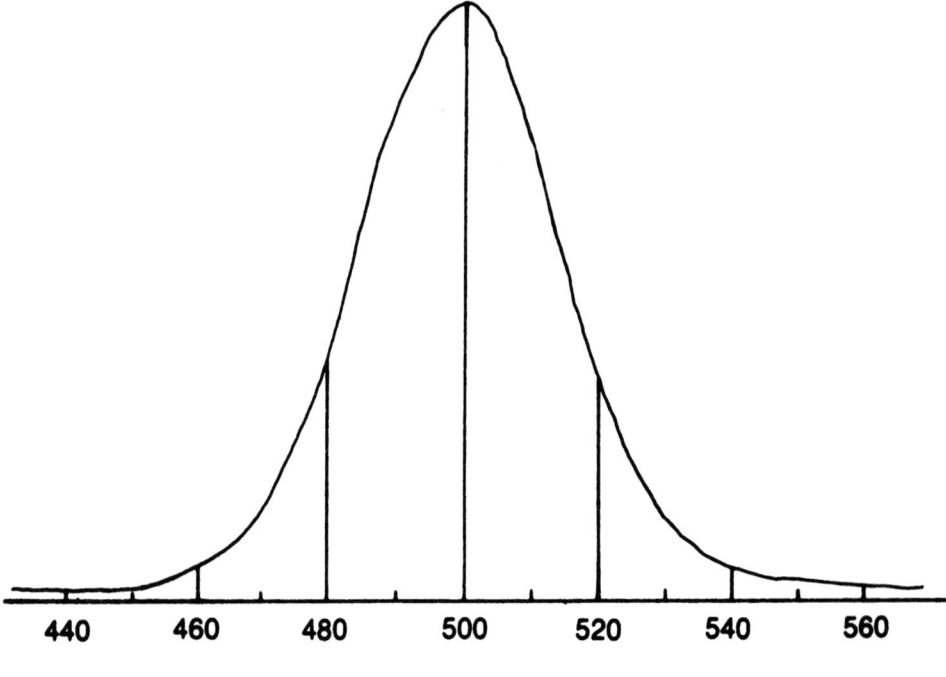

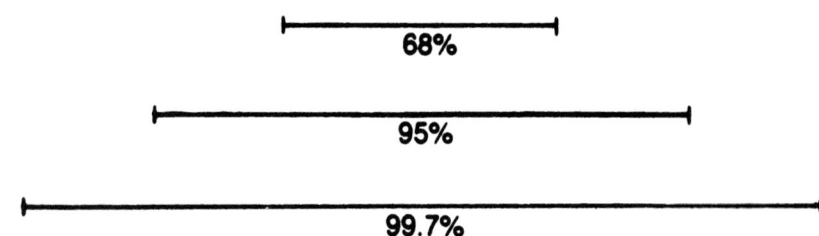

Figure 11–6. Sampling distribution

The actual situation is that the null hypothesis is:

		True	False
The researcher calculates a test statistic and decides that the null hypothesis is:	**True** (Null accepted)	Correct decision	Type II error
	False (Null rejected)	Type I error	Correct decision

Figure 11–7. Outcomes of statistical decision making

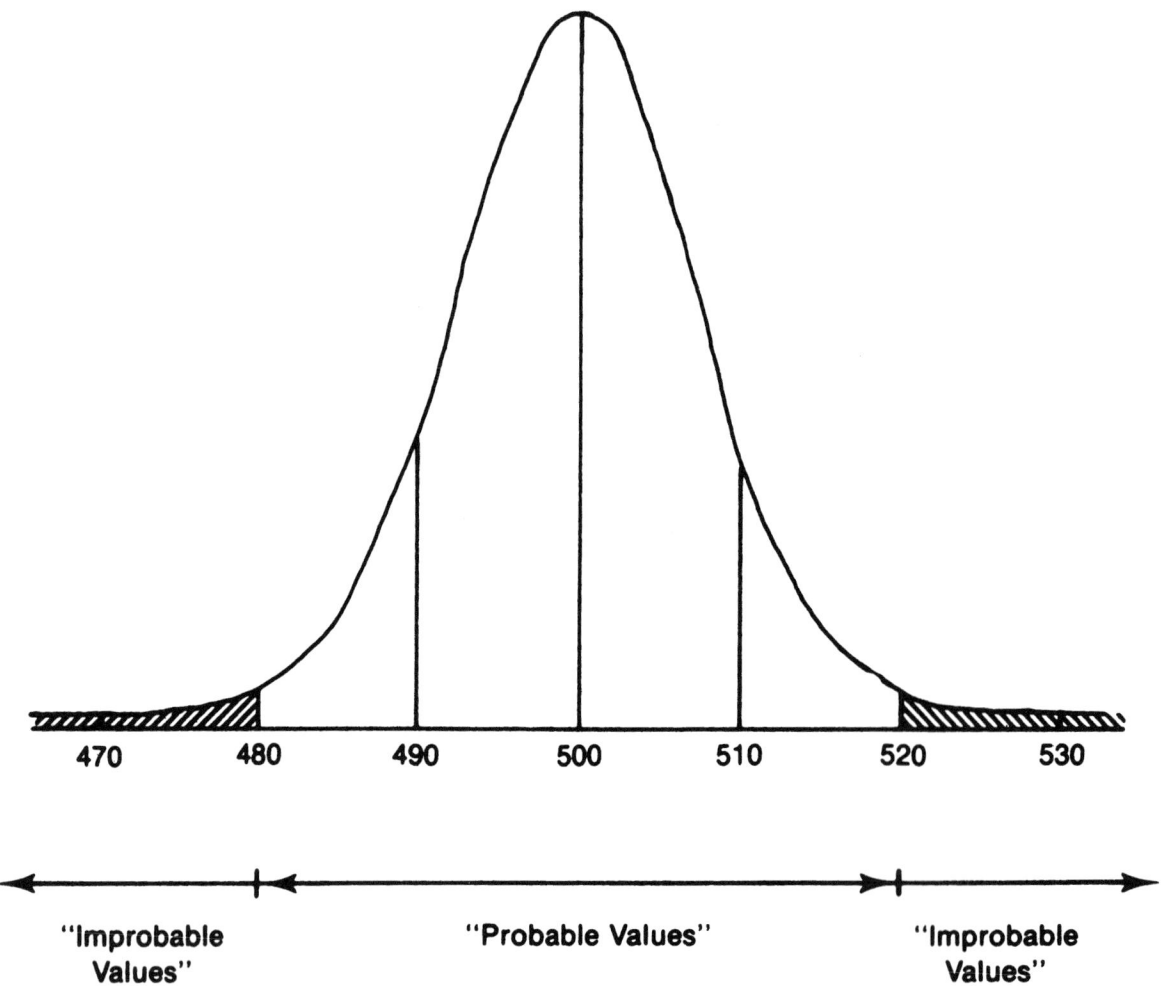

Figure 11–8. Sampling distribution for hypothesis test example

Table 11-15. Guide to Widely Used Bivariate Statistical Tests

Name	Test Statistic	Purpose	Measurement Level* IV	Measurement Level* DV
Parametric Tests				
t-test for independent groups	t	To test the difference between two independent group means	Nominal	Interval, Ratio
t-test for dependent groups	t	To test the difference between two dependent group means	Nominal	Interval, Ratio
Analysis of variance—ANOVA	F	To test the difference among the means of 3+ independent groups, or of more than one independent variable	Nominal	Interval, Ratio
Repeated measures ANOVA	F	To test the difference among means of 3+ related groups or sets of scores	Nominal	Interval, Ratio
Pearson's r	r	To test the existence of a relationship between two variables	Interval, Ratio	Interval, Ratio
Nonparametric Tests				
Chi-squared test	χ^2	To test the difference in proportions in 2+ independent groups	Nominal	Nominal
Mann-Whitney U-test	U	To test the difference in ranks of scores on two independent groups	Nominal	Ordinal
Kruskal-Wallis test	H	To test the difference in ranks of scores of 3+ independent groups	Nominal	Ordinal
Wilcoxon signed ranks test	$T\ (Z)$	To test the difference in ranks of scores of two related groups	Nominal	Ordinal
Friedman test	χ^2	To test the difference in ranks of scores of 3+ related groups	Nominal	Ordinal
Phi coefficient	ϕ	To test the magnitude of a relationship between two dichotomous variables	Nominal	Nominal
Spearman's rank order correlation	r_s	To test the existence of a relationship between two variables	Ordinal	Ordinal

*Measurement level of the independent variable (IV) and dependent variable (DV).

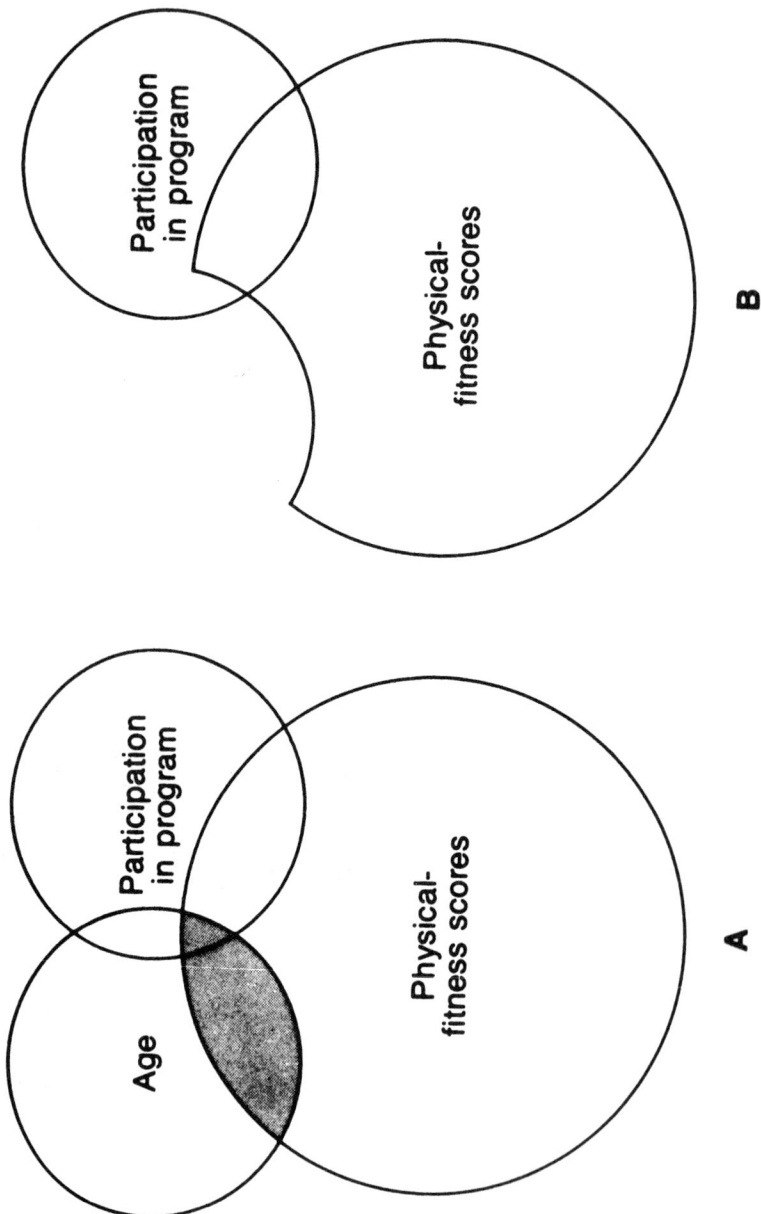

Figure 11–9. Schematic diagram illustrating the principle of analysis of covariance
Copyright © 1997 Lippincott-Raven Publishers
Polit/Hungler: Essentials of Nursing Research, fourth edition

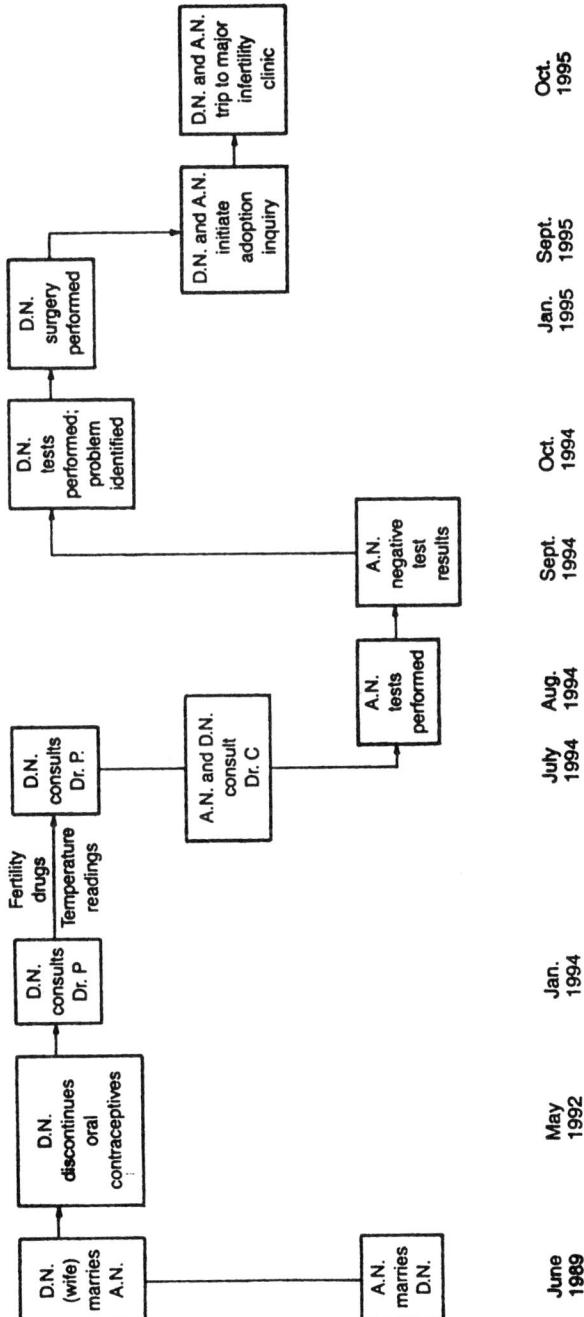

Figure 12–3. Example of a timeline for infertility study
Copyright © 1997 Lippincott-Raven Publishers
Polit/Hungler: Essentials of Nursing Research, fourth edition

POWER

+   −

The parents feel guilty despite professionals' attempts to eliminate guilt

Style is "committed"/"correcting the flaw"

The parents are especially "fused" to the child

Style is "stuck"/"secondary gains" or "protection from social responsibility"

The parents accept not feeling responsible and have power.

Style is "successful"/"mastery"

The parents accept not feeling responsible but let go of power.

Style is "letting go"/"new meaning"

+   −

RESPONSIBILITY

Figure 12–4. Barton's (1991) schema describing parental adaptation to adolescent drug abuse (Reprinted with permission)

Copyright © 1997 Lippincott-Raven Publishers
Polit/Hungler: Essentials of Nursing Research, fourth edition

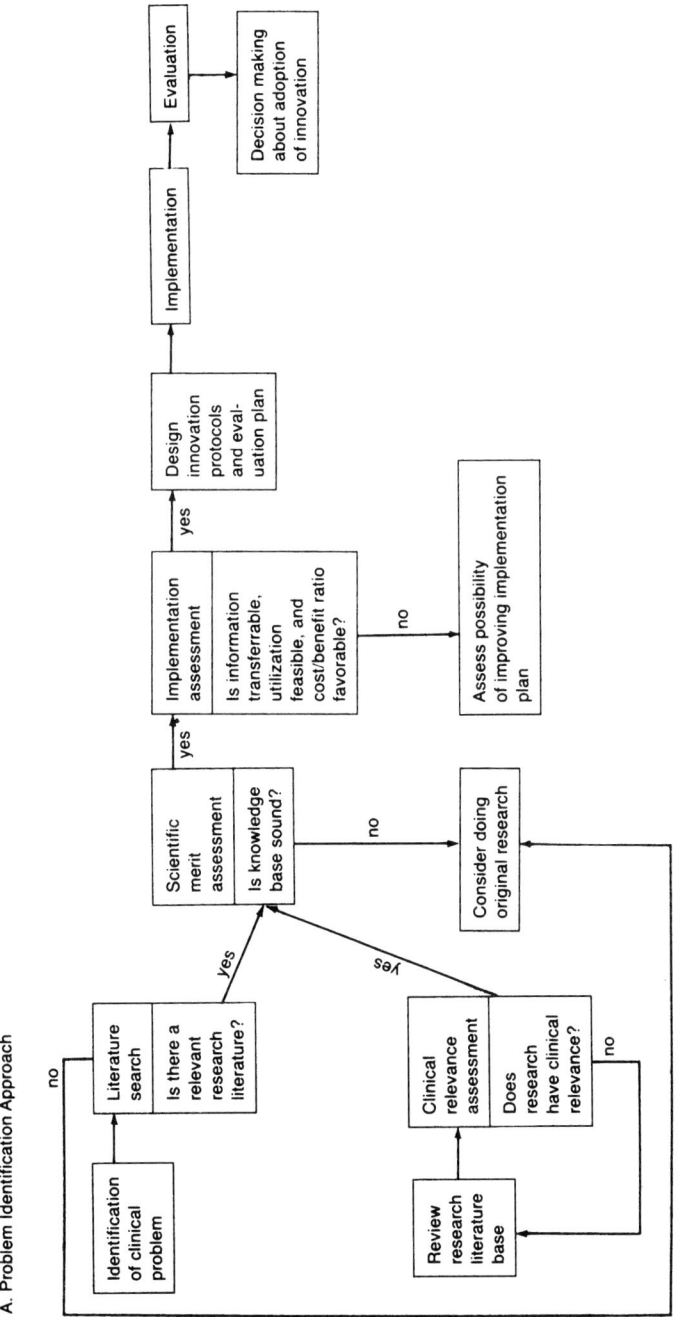

Figure 14–1. Two models of research utilization
Copyright © 1997 Lippincott-Raven Publishers
Polit/Hungler: Essentials of Nursing Research, fourth edition